Clinical Management of Chest Tubes

Editor

PIER LUIGI FILOSSO

THORACIC SURGERY CLINICS

www.thoracic.theclinics.com

Consulting Editor
M. BLAIR MARSHALL

February 2017 • Volume 27 • Number 1

ELSEVIER

1600 John F. Kennedy Boulevard • Suite 1800 • Philadelphia, Pennsylvania, 19103-2899

http://www.thoracic.theclinics.com

THORACIC SURGERY CLINICS Volume 27, Number 1
February 2017 ISSN 1547-4127, ISBN-13: 978-0-323-49679-7

Editor: John Vassallo (j.vassallo@elsevier.com)
Developmental Editor: Susan Showalter

Thoracic Surgery Clinics (ISSN 1547-4127) is published quarterly by Elsevier Inc., 360 Park Avenue South, New York, NY 10010-1710. Months of publication are February, May, August, and November. Business and editorial offices: 1600 John F. Kennedy Boulevard, Suite 1800, Philadelphia, PA 19103-2899. Periodicals postage paid at New York, NY, and additional mailing offices. Subscription prices are $359.00 per year (US individuals), $521.00 per year (US institutions), $100.00 per year (US Students), $439.00 per year (Canadian individuals), $674.00 per year (Canadian institutions), $225.00 per year (Canadian and international students), $470.00 per year (international individuals), and $674.00 per year (international institutions). Foreign air speed delivery is included in all Clinics' subscription prices. All prices are subject to change without notice. **POSTMASTER:** Send address changes to Thoracic Surgery Clinics, Elsevier Health Sciences Division, Subscription Customer Service, 3251 Riverport Lane, Maryland Heights, MO 63043. **Customer Service (orders, claims, online, change of address): Telephone: 1-800-654-2452 (U.S. and Canada); 314-447-8871 (outside U.S. and Canada). Fax: 314-447-8029. E-mail: journalscustomerservice-usa@elsevier.com (for print support); journalsonlinesupport-usa@elsevier.com (for online support).**

Reprints. For copies of 100 or more, of articles in this publication, please contact Commercial Rights Department, Elsevier Inc., 360 Park Avenue South, New York, NY 10010-1710. Tel: 212-633-3874; Fax: 212-633-3820; E-mail: reprints@elsevier.com.

Thoracic Surgery Clinics is covered in *MEDLINE/PubMed (Index Medicus)*, *EMBASE/Excerpta Medica*, *Science Citation Index Expanded (SciSearch®)*, *Journal Citation Reports/Science Edition,* and *Current Contents®/Clinical Medicine.*

Contributors

CONSULTING EDITOR

M. BLAIR MARSHALL, MD, FACS
Chief, Division of Thoracic Surgery; Associate
Professor of Surgery, Department of Surgery,
Georgetown University Medical Center,
Georgetown University School of Medicine,
Washington, DC

EDITOR

PIER LUIGI FILOSSO, MD, FECTS
Department of Thoracic Surgery, University of
Torino, Torino, Italy

AUTHORS

MARCO ANILE, MD
Department of Thoracic Surgery, Policlinico
Umberto I, University of Rome Sapienza,
Rome, Italy

LUCA ROSARIO ASSANTE, MD
Consultant Thoracic Endoscopist, Thoracic
Endoscopy Unit, Sacro Cuore Don Calabria
Research Hospital – Cancer Care Center,
Negrar, Verona, Italy

LUCA BERTOLACCINI, MD, PhD, FCCP
Consultant Thoracic Surgeon, Thoracic
Surgery Unit, Sacro Cuore Don Calabria
Research Hospital – Cancer Care Center,
Negrar, Verona, Italy

GIULIA BORA, MD
Department of Thoracic Surgery, University of
Torino, Torino, Italy

ALESSANDRO BRUNELLI, MD, FEBTS
Department of Thoracic Surgery, St. James's
University Hospital, Leeds, United Kingdom

DANIELE DISO, MD
Department of Thoracic Surgery, Policlinico
Umberto I, University of Rome Sapienza,
Rome, Italy

PIER LUIGI FILOSSO, MD, FECTS
Department of Thoracic Surgery, University of
Torino, Torino, Italy

FRANCESCO GUERRERA, MD
Department of Thoracic Surgery, University of
Torino, Torino, Italy

MARCELO F. JIMÉNEZ, MD, PhD, EBCTS
Professor, General Thoracic Surgery Service,
University Hospital of Salamanca, Salamanca,
Spain

ERIC LIM, MBChB, MD, MSc, FRCS(C-Th)
Department of Cardiothoracic Surgery, James
Cook University Hospital, Middlesbrough;
Imperial College and the Academic Division of
Thoracic Surgery, Royal Brompton Hospital,
London, United Kingdom

PHILIP J. McELNAY, MBChB, MRCS
Department of Cardiothoracic Surgery, James
Cook University Hospital, Middlesbrough,
United Kingdom

TAMAS F. MOLNAR, MD, PhD, DSc, FETS
Professor of Surgery; Department of
Operational Medicine, Faculty of Medicine,
University of Pécs, Pécs, Hungary; Thoracic
Surgery Unit, Department of Surgery, Aladar
Petz Teaching Hospital, Győr, Hungary

NURIA M. NOVOA, MD, PhD
Associated Professor, General Thoracic
Surgery Service, University Hospital of
Salamanca, Salamanca, Spain

ALBERTO OLIARO, MD
Department of Thoracic Surgery, University of
Torino, Torino, Italy

ILARIA ONORATI, MD
Department of Thoracic Surgery, Policlinico
Umberto I, University of Rome Sapienza,
Rome, Italy

SIMONA PAIANO, MD
Consultant Thoracic Endoscopist, Thoracic
Endoscopy Unit, Sacro Cuore Don Calabria
Research Hospital – Cancer Care Center,
Negrar, Verona, Italy

CARLO POMARI, MD
Chief, Thoracic Endoscopy Unit, Sacro Cuore
Don Calabria Research Hospital – Cancer Care
Center, Negrar, Verona, Italy

CECILIA POMPILI, MD
Department of Thoracic Surgery, St. James's
University Hospital, Leeds, United Kingdom

ERINO A. RENDINA, MD
Department of Thoracic Surgery, University of
Rome Sapienza, Ospedale S.Andrea, Rome,
Italy

GAETANO ROCCO, MD, FRCSEd, FEBTS
Division of Thoracic Surgical Oncology,
Department of Thoracic Surgical and Medical
Oncology, Istituto Nazionale Tumori, Pascale
Foundation, IRCCS, Naples, Italy

RAFFAELE ROCCO, MD
Section of Thoracic Surgery, University
Campus Biomedico, Rome, Italy

MATTEO ROFFINELLA, MD
Department of Thoracic Surgery, University of
Torino, Torino, Italy

ENRICO RUFFINI, MD, FECTS
Department of Thoracic Surgery, University of
Torino, Torino, Italy

MICHELE SALATI, MD
Division of Thoracic Surgery, Ospedali Riuniti,
Ancona, Italy

ALBERTO SANDRI, MD
Department of Thoracic Surgery, University of
Torino, Torino, Italy

PAOLO SOLIDORO, MD
Unit of Pulmonology, San Giovanni Battista
Hospital, Torino, Italy

ALBERTO TERZI, MD
Chief, Thoracic Surgery Unit, Sacro Cuore Don
Calabria Research Hospital – Cancer Care
Center, Negrar, Verona, Italy

GONZALO VARELA, MD, PhD, EBCTS
Professor, General Thoracic Surgery Service,
University Hospital of Salamanca, Salamanca,
Spain

FEDERICO VENUTA, MD
Cattedra di Chirurgia Toracica, Department of
Thoracic Surgery, Policlinico Umberto I,
University of Rome Sapienza, Rome, Italy

ANDREA VITI, MD, PhD
Consultant Thoracic Surgeon, Thoracic
Surgery Unit, Sacro Cuore Don Calabria
Research Hospital – Cancer Care Center,
Negrar, Verona, Italy

Contents

Federico Venuta, Daniele Diso, Marco Anile, Erino A. Rendina, and Ilaria Onorati

Insertion, management, and withdrawal of chest tubes is part of the routine activity of thoracic surgeons. The selection of the chest tube and the strategy for each of these steps is usually built on knowledge, practice, experience, and judgment. The indication to insert a chest tube into the pleural cavity is the presence of air or fluid within it. Various types and sizes of chest tubes are now commercially available.

Pier Luigi Filosso, Alberto Sandri, Francesco Guerrera, Matteo Roffinella, Giulia Bora, and Paolo Solidoro

Immediately after lung resection, air tends to collect in the retrosternal part of the chest wall (in supine position), and fluids in its lower part (costodiaphragmatic sinus). Several general thoracic surgery textbooks currently recommend the placement of 2 chest tubes after major pulmonary resections, one anteriorly, to remove air, and another into the posterior and basilar region, to drain fluids. Recently, several authors advocated the placement of a single chest tube. In terms of air and fluid drainage, this technique demonstrated to be as effective as the conventional one after wedge resection or uncomplicated lobectomy.

Tamas F. Molnar

Clinical suspicion of hemo/pneumothorax: when in doubt, drain the chest. Stable chest trauma with hemo/pneumothorax: drain and wait. Unstable patient with dislocated trachea must be approached with drain in hand and scalpel ready. Massive hemo/pneumothorax may be controlled by drainage alone. The surgeon should not hesitate to open the chest if too much blood drains over a short period. The chest drainage procedure does not end with the last stitch; the second half of the match is still ahead. The drained patient is in need of physiotherapy and proper pain relief with an extended pleural space: control the suction system.

Cecilia Pompili, Michele Salati, and Alessandro Brunelli

There is scant evidence on the management of chest tubes after surgery for pneumothorax. Most of the current knowledge is extrapolated from studies performed on subjects with lung cancer. This article reviews the existing literature with particular focus on the effect of suction and no suction on the duration of air leak after lung resection and surgery for pneumothorax. Moreover, the role of regulated suction, which seems to provide some benefit in reducing pneumothorax recurrence after bullectomy and pleurodesis, is discussed. Finally, a personal view on the management of chest tubes after surgery for pneumothorax is provided.

Both physicians and surgeons insert chest drains by various techniques—including Seldinger and "wide-bore" methods. The indications include hemothorax, pneumothorax, pleural effusion, and postoperative care in thoracic surgery. Given their invasive nature, there is significant potential for complications; however, this can be minimized by following a meticulous technique, which is herein described for both Seldinger and "wide-bore" drain insertion.

Despite several randomized trials and meta-analyses, the dilemma as to whether to apply suction after subtotal pulmonary resection has not been solved. The combination of a poorly understood pathophysiology of the air leak phenomenon and the inadequate quality of the published randomized trials is actually preventing thoracic surgeons from abandoning an empirical management of chest drains. Even digital systems do not seem to have made the difference so far. Based on the evidence of the literature, the authors propose a new air leak predictor score (ALPS) as a contributing step toward appropriateness in using intraoperative sealants, opting for an external suction and managing and chest tubes.

Despite the increasing knowledge about the pleural physiology after lung resection, most practices around chest tube removal are dictated by personal preferences and experience. This article discusses recently published data on the topic and suggests opportunities for further investigation and future improvements.

Malignant pleural effusion (MPE) symptoms have a real impact on quality of life. Surgical approach through video-assisted thoracic surgery provides a first step in palliation. In patients unfit for general anesthesia, awake pleuroscopy represents an alternative. Sclerosing agents can be administered at the bedside through a chest tube. Ideal treatment of MPE should include adequate long-term symptom relief, minimize hospitalization, and reduce adverse effects. Indwelling pleural catheter (IPC) allows outpatient management of MPE through periodic ambulatory fluid drainage. IPC offers advantages over pleurodesis in patients with poor functional status who cannot tolerate pleurodesis or in patients with trapped lungs.

Chest drain placement is one of the most common surgical procedures performed in routine clinical practice. Despite the many benefits, chest tube insertion is not always a harmless procedure, and potential significant morbidity and mortality may exist. The aim of this article was to highlight the correct chest tube placement procedure and to focus on errors and clinical complications following its incorrect insertion into the chest.

THORACIC SURGERY CLINICS

THE CLINICS ARE AVAILABLE ONLINE!
Access your subscription at:
www.theclinics.com

Preface
Chest Drainage Management: Where Are We Now?

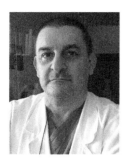

Pier Luigi Filosso, MD, FECTS
Editor

This issue of *Thoracic Surgery Clinics* is dedicated to the management of chest drains.

Chest drain insertion is one of the most common surgical procedures performed in routine clinical practice. It is usually performed by thoracic surgeons but, oftentimes, also by emergency physicians, intensivists, pulmonologists, interventional radiologists, and nonphysician advanced practitioners in the emergency setting. Despite the many benefits, this procedure is not devoid of complications, and potential significant morbidity and mortality may exist. Furthermore, its management is usually strictly dependent on the physician's personal preference, since up to now, univocal guidelines did not exist.

This issue's review articles cover most of what physicians face when treating a patient with a chest tube, and have been written by world-renowned experts in this field.

I am deeply indebted to all of the authors who contributed to the realization of this issue, as well as the Elsevier staff, particularly John Vassallo and Susan Showalter, with whom I had long discussions that helped me in the finalization of this issue.

Finally, I wish to dedicate this issue of *Thoracic Surgery Clinics* to all those women and men surgeons who, through their hard work, daily commitment, and devotion to the field of thoracic surgery help to promote and progress our specialty, ensuring patients a high quality of care and a better quality of life, and improving their long-term survival.

Pier Luigi Filosso, MD, FECTS
University of Torino
Department of Thoracic Surgery
C.so Dogliotti 14
Torino 10126, Italy

E-mail address:
pierluigi.filosso@unito.it

Thorac Surg Clin 27 (2017) ix
http://dx.doi.org/10.1016/j.thorsurg.2016.10.001
1547-4127/17/© 2016 Published by Elsevier Inc.

Chest Tubes: Generalities

Federico Venuta, MD[a,*], Daniele Diso, MD[a], Marco Anile, MD[a],
Erino A. Rendina, MD[b], Ilaria Onorati, MD[a]

KEYWORDS

- Chest drainage • Chest tube • Air leak • Pleural effusions • Pneumothorax

KEY POINTS

- Insertion, management, and withdrawal of chest tubes is part of the routine activity of thoracic surgeons.
- The selection of the chest tube and the strategy for each of these steps is usually built on knowledge, practice, experience, and judgment.
- The indication to insert a chest tube into the pleural cavity is the presence of air or fluid within it.
- Various types and sizes of chest tubes are now commercially available.

Insertion, management, and withdrawal of chest tubes is part of the routine activity of thoracic surgeons. The selection of the chest tube and the strategy for each of these steps is usually built on knowledge, practice, experience, and judgment. The indication to insert a chest tube into the pleural cavity is the presence of air or fluid within it. The goals should be:

- To evacuate air or fluid from the pleural space
- To collapse any residual cavity in order to prevent subsequent pleural problems
- To ensure complete pulmonary reexpansion and restore respiratory mechanics

The achievement of these goals depends on:

- Viscosity of the pleural fluid and presence of debris within it
- Whether the fluid is uniloculated or multiloculated
- Size of the underlying/residual lung
- Capability of the underlying/residual lung to reexpand and occupy the pleural space
- Presence of air leaks (both alveolar or bronchopleural fistula)

HISTORY

Hippocrates was the first to drain the pleural space: he described incision, cautery, and metal tubes to drain empyemas.[1] Hunter, in the 1860s, developed a hypodermic needle and inserted it into the pleural space for drainage purposes.[2] Continuous chest tube drainage of the pleural space incorporating an underwater seal device seems to have been first performed by Playfair[3] in the 1870s in a patient with empyema unresponsive to repeated aspiration. Hewett[4] described closed tube drainage of an empyema in 1876. However, extensive use of this technique was not reported until 1917, when it was successfully used to drain postinfluenza epidemic empyemas.[5]

The use of chest tubes to drain the chest cavity after thoracic surgery procedures was reported by Lilienthal[6] in 1922; this included lobectomy for suppurative diseases. It was not until the Korean War that postoperative chest tube placement became the gold standard after major thoracic surgery procedures.[7] As a consequence, the use of closed systems became more popular than open drainage systems (rib resection with open drainage or Eloesser flap). The mortality for empyema treated with rib resection and leaving the chest open was 28%, compared with 4% for closed pleural drainage.[8]

Gotthard Bulau, a German internist, is credited as the first to design a closed water seal drainage system.[9,10] Based on these findings, closed

Conflicts of Interest: The authors have no related conflict of interest to declare.
[a] Department of Thoracic Surgery, Policlinico Umberto I, University of Rome Sapienza, V.le del Policlinico, Rome, Italy; [b] Department of Thoracic Surgery, University of Rome Sapienza, Ospedale S.Andrea, Rome, Italy
* Corresponding author.
E-mail address: federico.venuta@uniroma1.it

thoracic.theclinics.com

pleural space drainage became the standard of care in the early twentieth century and it is part of the modern era of thoracic surgery. Chest tubes made of several different materials in different designs and sizes have been produced and have been accompanied by the development of different pleural drainage units.

AIR AND FLUID ACCUMULATION IN THE PLEURAL SPACE

Gas and fluid, when profuse, can completely fill the pleural space; in contrast, smaller amounts of fluid may collect only in selected areas based on its nature and density, the quality of the underlying lung and visceral pleura, and the presence of pleural adhesions.

Air tends to collect in the upper part of the chest. Fluids tend to accumulate in the lower part of the chest cavity, which is inferior in the sitting or standing position, or posterior with the patient supine (costophrenic and costovertebral spaces, respectively).

These variables are crucial to choose the optimal site for tube drainage both of a free pleural space and a multiloculated effusion. Particularly, the latter situation requires precise localization of chest radiograph and computed tomography (CT) scan.

INDICATIONS FOR CHEST TUBE PLACEMENT

Indications for chest tube insertion are the following:

- Pneumothorax (according to guidelines)
- Penetrating chest injuries
- Hemopneumothorax
- Recurrent symptomatic pleural effusions
- Empyema and parapneumonic effusions
- Chylothorax
- Postoperatively in thoracic and cardiac surgery
- Bronchopleural fistula

Absolute contraindications do not exist; coagulopathies and platelet defects require specific considerations on a case-by-case basis with correction of the disorder if patient stability allows it.[11] Chest tube insertion in a skin area with benign or malignant disorders should be avoided if possible.

CHEST TUBE PLACEMENT, MANAGEMENT, AND REMOVAL

The site of chest tube insertion is usually determined by the material that requires drainage and the location within the pleural space. Insertion is guided by chest radiograph or CT scan when available. Ultrasonography can also be useful, particularly in intensive care patients who cannot be moved to more sophisticated radiological equipment or when lateral projections cannot be recorded. Chest tubes can be inserted in the midaxillary line at the level of the third or fifth intercostal space. Alternatively, the second intercostal space on the midclavicular line can be chosen, particularly in cases of small apical pneumothorax. However, also in these cases, the authors prefer the fifth intercostal space on the lateral side of the chest, pushing the tube as far up as possible. Insertion of the chest tube should be preceded by local anesthesia and careful maneuvers should avoid injuring the intercostal vessels and nerve, staying as close as possible to the border of the lower rib of the space. Aspiration of air or fluid into the anesthetic syringe indicates entrance in the pleural space. Blunt dissection and finger exploration should be encouraged to avoid injuring the lung parenchyma. The chest tube should be sewn in place using heavy suture material (0 silk). Placement of an additional purse string suture at this time, under the effect of local anesthesia, helps at the time of chest tube removal. Chest radiograph after placement of thoracic drainage is mandatory. It helps to confirm the correct position of the tube; if the tube requires repositioning, this can be done with local anesthesia still active.

In difficult situations, small-bore chest tubes can be placed under CT guidance with the Seldinger technique.

At the end of a surgical procedure 1 or 2 chest tubes are placed under direct visual control. If 2 chest tubes are placed the posterior is left lower in the chest cage to drain blood, whereas the anterior is pulled up to the apex to drain air. If only 1 chest tube is inserted, this is usually located posteriorly and pulled up the apex of the chest. Additional holes are made to drain fluids from the lower part of the thoracic cavity.

The size of the chest tube should be based on the type of intrathoracic collection that requires drainage. Small-bore catheters are used with an increased frequency in cases of pneumothorax. In contrast, empyema always requires large-bore tubes because of the viscosity of pus.

Various types and sizes of tubes are currently available. The key factor in selecting the correct size of tube is the air or liquid flow rate that can be obtained through the tube. This rate is determined by the Fanning equation:

$$v = \pi^2 r^5 p/fl$$

where v is the flow, r is the radius of the tube, p is the pressure, f is the friction factor, and l is the length.[12,13] Thus, the inner bore of the tube and its length are crucial. However, no single formula can be used because of the variety of liquids and accompanying fluid debris that may be drained from the chest. The selection of the chest tube size must also take into account the rate of production of the fluid or the amount of air leak. The production of more viscous fluids, like blood or pus, requires larger-bore tubes compared with when a similar volume of air is produced.[14]

Minor complications of chest tube placement include patient discomfort during tube insertion, residence, and removal; misplacement of the tube during insertion; disconnection of the tube and leakage around the tube; and that, if the last hole of the tube is not completely within the chest, subcutaneous emphysema may be observed. Major complications include laceration of the lung parenchyma or diaphragm, and even the liver (particularly in patients with ascites or cirrhosis), and bleeding from an intercostal vessel. Colonization and infection of the site of insertion, particularly if the tube is left in place for a long time, may also be observed.

Chest tubes should be removed after careful assessment of the clinical status of the patient and chest radiograph viewing. Chest tubes are usually removed after asking the patient to take a deep breath and hold it as the tube is removed; the site is then covered and taped. Suction should be applied during removal. If 2 chest tubes are in place, the first to be removed is the posterior-lower one. This system allows the upper-anterior tube to drain air if it enters during the removal maneuver.

In case of prolonged air leaks, the chest tube can be removed after provocative chest tube clamping.[15] The safety of this technique is probably related to the development of adhesions as a result of surgical maneuvers and chest tube placement. These adhesions prevent pneumothorax from developing because the rest of the lung is stuck, although part of it is still leaking.

Management of chest drainage is still debated. Most surgeons still apply suction, especially after lung surgery. Suction is thought to improve reexpansion of the residual lung and drainage of fluids. However, 63% of the surgeons participating in a Society of Thoracic Surgeons survey put the chest tubes on water seal for 12 to 24 hours before removing them in the absence of air leaks.[16]

Once the chest tube is in place, a pleural drainage unit is usually attached to provide suction or a water seal to prevent the backflow of air into the pleura space. A 1-way valve is essential whenever there is the possibility of air leaks; it allows air to exit along a low-resistance path, preserving negative pleural pressure and permitting lung reexpansion. The basic original drainage system is the 3-bottle system. This system allows the application of suction through the third bottle and, most important, it allows the fluid (blood) to drain into the first bottle only while air escapes into the second bottle. This system prevents foam from forming in the first bottle.

The appropriate use of pleural drainage systems for pneumothorax has been reported by the American College of Chest Physicians (ACCP),[17] but it is less defined for traumatic or iatrogenic pneumothorax.[14] Pleural and free-flowing fluids generally drain out of the chest through the chest drainage without the need of suction. The ACCP guidelines for pneumothorax treatment suggest that both suction and nonsuction are acceptable[17]; if gravity water seal drainage is not effective, suction can be applied.

The decision to apply suction after general thoracic procedures is more controversial. Suction should speed the removal of air and fluid from the intrathoracic cavity; this should contribute to avoiding residual spaces and favor complete reexpansion of the lung. However, notwithstanding these obvious advantages, some surgeons are in favor but others strongly believe that suction contributes to prolonging air leaks.[18]

This topic was investigated by Sanni and colleagues[19] in 2006; out of 6 studies in the international literature, none reported that suction was able to reduce air leaks, 2 found no difference, and 4 concluded that application of suction postoperatively increased the incidence of air leaks. Two meta-analysis were published in 2010 and 2012[20,21]; both concluded that there were no differences in terms of occurrence of prolonged air leaks, duration of air leaks, chest tube duration, and length of hospital stay if suction was applied or not postoperatively. These findings were subsequently confirmed by a recent analysis[22]: suction hastens the removal of air and fluid but does not offer improved clinical outcomes. However, the application of suction significantly reduced the occurrence of postoperative pneumothorax. In that study, a national survey showed that 68% of surgeons routinely apply low-pressure suction to the drains after lung resections (nonpneumonectomy).

The Heimlich valve is an example of a passive system that allows mobilization and even discharge of the patient without discomfort.

Commercially available pleural drainage units have been compared in terms of flow rates and pressures generated.[23] Differences have been recorded regarding both variables; the investigators suggest that differences in flow rates may be clinically important in patients with air leaks related to large pneumothoraces; differences in generated pressures are likely not clinically important.

Digital pleural drainage systems have recently been commercialized. These systems have a screen where instantaneous values of pleural pressure and flow are shown or their temporal trends can be displayed; these data can be downloaded on a computer and subsequently analyzed.[24] Some companies also provide commercialized systems with a stand-alone suction pump, allowing them to be carried around and giving the patient the freedom to ambulate without being attached to wall suction. The use of these systems contributes to shortening hospital stay by leading to earlier chest tube removal in patients with air leaks.[24] Furthermore, patients can be discharged home with these devices in place, given the absence of contraindications patients have to remain within an appropriate distance from medical support, have reasonable pain control, and not have marginal pulmonary function.[25–27]

REFERENCES

1. Hutchins RA. Hippocrates, writings. In: Great books of the Western world, vol. 29. Chicago: Encyclopedia Britannica; 1952. p. 142.
2. Hochberg LA. Thoracic surgery before the twentieth century. New York: Vantage Press; 1960. p. 255.
3. Playfair GE. Case of empyema treated by aspiration and subsequently by drainage: recovery. Br Med J 1875;1:45.
4. Hewett C. Drainage for empyema treated by aspiration. Br Med J 1876;1:317.
5. Graham EA, Bell RD. Open pneumothorax: its relation to the treatment of empyema. Am J Med Sci 1918;156:839–71.
6. Lilienthal H. Resection of the lung for suppurative infections with a report based on 31 consecutive operative cases in which resection was done or intended. Ann Surg 1922;75:257–320.
7. Lawrance GH. Closed chest tube drainage for pleural space problems. In: Major problems in clinical surgery. Problems of the pleural space, vol. 28. 1983. p. 14–24.
8. Cerfolio RJ. Closed drainage and suction systems. In: Patterson GA, editor. Pearson's thoracic & esophageal surgery. Philadelphia: Churchill Livingstone – Elsevier; 2008. p. 1147–54.
9. Meyer JA. Gotthard Bulau and closed water seal drainage for empyema, 1875 – 1891. Ann Thorac Surg 1989;48:597–9.
10. Van Schil PE. Thoracic drainage and the contribution of Gotthard Bulau. Ann Thorac Surg 1997;63:1876.
11. Baumann MH, Strange C. The clinician's perspective on pneumothorax management. Chest 1997;112:822–8.
12. Baumann MH, Strange C. Treatment of spontaneous pneumothorax. A more aggressive approach? Chest 1997;112:789–804.
13. Swenson EW, Birath G, Ahbeck A. Resistance to air flow in bronchospirometric catheters. J Thorac Surg 1957;33:275–81.
14. Baumann MH. What size of chest tube? What drainage system is ideal? And other chest tube management questions. Curr Opin Pulm Med 2003;9:276–81.
15. Kirschner PA. Provocative clamping and removal of chest tube despite patient air leak. Ann Thorac Surg 1992;53:740–1.
16. Kim SS, Khalpey Z, Daugherty SL, et al. Factors in the selection and management of chest tubes after pulmonary lobectomy: results of a national survey of thoracic surgeons. Ann Thorac Surg 2016;101:1082–8.
17. Baumann MH, Strange C, Heffner JE, et al. Management of spontaneous pneumothorax. An American College of Chest Physicians Delphi Consensus Statement. Chest 2001;119:590–602.
18. Alphonso N, Tan C, Utely M, et al. A prospective randomized controlled trial of suction versus non suction to the underwater seal drains following lung resection. Eur J Cardiothorac Surg 2005;27:391–4.
19. Sanni S, Critcly A, Dunning J. Should chest drains be put on suction or not following pulmonary lobectomy? Interact Cardiovasc Thorac Surg 2006;5:275–8.
20. Deng B, Tan QY, Zhao YP, et al. Suction or non-suction to the underwater seal drains following pulmonary operation: meta-analysis of randomized controlled trials. Eur J Cardiothorac Surg 2010;38:210–5.
21. Coughlan SM, Emmerton-Coughlin HMA, Maltheiner R. Management of chest tubes after pulmonary resection: a systematic review and meta-analysis. Can J Surg 2012;55:264–70.
22. Lang P, Manickavasagar M, Burdett C, et al. Suction of chest drains following lung resection: evidence and practice are not aligned. Eur J Cardiothorac Surg 2016;49:611–6.
23. Baumann MH, Patel PB, Roney CW, et al. Comparison of function of commonly available pleural drainage units and catheters. Chest 2003;123:1878–86.
24. Cerfolio RJ, Varela G, Brunelli A. Digital and smart chest drainage systems to monitor air leaks: the birth of a new era? Thorac Surg Clin 2010;20:413–20.

25. Varela G, Jimenez MF, Novoa N. Portable chest drainage systems and outpatient chest tube management. Thorac Surg Clin 2010;20:421–6.
26. Rieger KM, Wroblewski HA, Brooks JA, et al. Postoperative outpatient chest tube management: initial experience with a portable system. Ann Thorac Surg 2007;84:630–2.
27. Cerfolio RJ, Minnich DJ, Bryant AS. The removal of chest tubes despite an air leak or a pneumothorax. Ann Thorac Surg 2009;87:1690–6.

Management of Chest Drains After Thoracic Resections

Pier Luigi Filosso, MD, FECTS[a],*, Alberto Sandri, MD[a],
Francesco Guerrera, MD[a], Matteo Roffinella, MD[a],
Giulia Bora, MD[a], Paolo Solidoro, MD[b]

KEYWORDS

• Pleura • Pleural fluid • Chest drain • Pulmonary resection • Postoperative course

KEY POINTS

• Immediately after lung resection, air tends to collect in the retrosternal part of the chest wall (in supine position), and fluids in its lower part (costodiaphragmatic sinus).
• Several general thoracic surgery textbooks currently recommend the placement of 2 chest tubes after major pulmonary resections, one anteriorly, to remove air, and another into the posterior and basilar region, to drain fluids.
• Recently, several authors advocated the placement of a single chest tube. In terms of air and fluid drainage, this technique demonstrated to be as effective as the conventional one after wedge resection or uncomplicated lobectomy.
• A single chest tube is less painful than 2 and, therefore, patients are able to perform postoperative respiratory physiotherapy adequately; this reflects on a better lung expansion, decreasing the risk of possible respiratory complications.

PLEURAL PHYSIOLOGY PILLS

The pleural space is a perfect biological system capable of accomplishing at least 2 fundamental functions: (1) to maintain the lung perfectly expanded in the chest, and (2) to preserve a perfect sliding between visceral and parietal pleura, with a very low coefficient of friction. Pleural fluid is kept in a subatmospheric range, which results by balancing its filtration and drainage.[1]

From an anatomic point of view, the pleural space is delimited by the visceral pleura, which wraps the entire lung and the fissures, and the parietal one, which covers the rib cage along with the diaphragmatic surface. Also, the parietal pleura is rich in lymphatics, that directly opens on the mesothelial surface trough the lymphatic stomata.[2,3] On the other hand, visceral pleura's lymphatics do not connect directly with the pleural space and therefore are not involved in the drainage of the pleural fluid.

The pleural fluid is hypo-oncotic (~ 1 g/dL protein),[4] explaining the low permeability of the parietal pleura to water and proteins. The overall pleural fluid turnover is estimated to be ~ 0.15 mL/kg/h.[4] In physiologic conditions, the pleural liquid pressure (P_{liq}) is more subatmospheric, while increasing the height in the pleural cavity, being about 0 at the bottom and ~ 10 cm H_2O at the midheart level. The role of pleural lymphatics is therefore paramount to (1) set a P_{liq} capable to maintain lung and chest wall together; (2) act as a regulator of pleural fluid volume, balancing its drainage and filtration. Whenever the lymphatic drainage becomes inefficient, pleural

[a] Department of Thoracic Surgery, University of Torino, Corso Dogliotti 14, Torino 10126, Italy; [b] Unit of Pulmonology, San Giovanni Battista Hospital, Via Genova 3, Torino 10126, Italy
* Corresponding author.
E-mail address: pierluigi.filosso@unito.it

Thorac Surg Clin 27 (2017) 7–11
http://dx.doi.org/10.1016/j.thorsurg.2016.08.002

fluid starts to accumulate in the pleural cavity, determining lung collapse.

As a consequence of pulmonary resections, the mechanical and pleural characteristics alter, even after the chest closure. The immediate problem after a thoracic operation is the correct evacuation of air from the cavity, accumulated as a consequence of the surgical maneuvers. Furthermore, a smaller lung must fill up the pleural cavity, which previously hosted a larger one: the compliance of the remaining part of the lung parenchyma appears to be decreased, correlated to the amount of the resected lung as well as to the intrinsic lung tissue characteristics. The remaining lung re-expansion requires a considerable lower subatmospheric P_{liq} along with a deformation of its natural shape. Furthermore, removing air from the chest wall results in the overdistension of unresected lung alveoli, which may favor persistent air leak and may be the cause of possible pulmonary edema.[5] A severe perturbation of the lung-water balance is also a major cause of developing other postresectional complications, such as atelectasis, acute lung injury, and acute respiratory distress syndrome.[6,7]

Immediately after lung resection, air tends to collect in the retrosternal part of the chest wall (in supine position), whereas fluids are located in its lower part (costodiaphragmatic sinus).[8,9] This condition explains why some surgeons use 2 drains after pulmonary resections, whereas some others prefer a single chest tube, to drain both air and fluids.

Air and fluid drainage may be increased by the use of an active suction, but the most innovative technique in chest drainage management is the adoption of a "controlled drainage," capable of avoiding an immediate lung overdistension, which may represent one of the major causes of postoperative development of complications.

NUMBER, TYPE, AND SIZE OF CHEST TUBES

Management of chest tubes after lung resection is still determined by the surgeons' habit and personal experience rather than valid scientific evidence. Moreover, chest tube duration is one of the most important factors influencing the overall hospital length of stay, hospitalization costs, as well as morbidity in general. Many textbooks recommend that, after a lobectomy, the pleural space should be drained by 2 chest tubes placed at the end of the surgical procedure: one in the anterior region, to remove air, and another in the posterior and basilar region, to drain fluids[10] (Fig. 1). Furthermore, according to a recent survey of thoracic surgery practice in the United

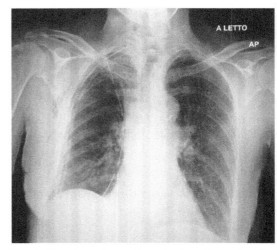

Fig. 1. Day 1 postoperative chest radiograph after right upper sleeve lobectomy: 2 chest drains (one anterior, another posterior) have been placed at the end of the intervention. The lung is correctly re-expanded.

Kingdom, more than 90% of thoracic surgeons leave 2 drains after both anatomic and nonanatomic lung resections.[11]

An inadequate residual lung re-expansion (Fig. 2) may also result in possible severe complications, such as atelectasis, hemothorax, or persistent air leak. From the mere physics point of view, the chest drain's effectiveness mostly depends on its diameter, and therefore, a large-bore chest tube (24 Fr–32 Fr) is advocated. However, small-bore drains have been recently used for the drainage of spontaneous pneumothorax or malignant pleural effusions,[12,13] but actually, to date, no scientific evidence related to their

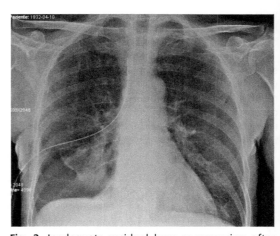

Fig. 2. Inadequate residual lung re-expansion after right lower lobectomy.

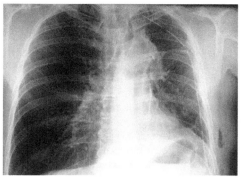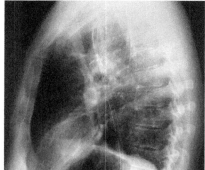

Fig. 3. Postoperative chest radiograph of a single chest drain (28-Fr Argyle) after left upper lobectomy.

effectiveness after pulmonary resections has been published.

More recently, several papers demonstrated that following wedge resection or lobectomy, a single chest drain (**Fig. 3**) is as effective as using the conventional two[14,15]; theoretically, a single chest drain causes less pain and discomfort to the patient compared with 2 tubes, and this may be translated into an improvement of patient's postoperative physiotherapy, which in turn may facilitate a better lung expansion, thus decreasing the risk of possible respiratory complications. An early patient discharge from the hospital is also achieved by this technique.

A recent meta-analysis[16] pooling data from a large number of patients treated and published in the previous studies confirmed that (1) one chest tube after lobectomy is less painful than 2 (95% confidence interval [CI]: 0.52–0.68, $P<.00001$); (2) a single drain was removed sooner (95% CI: 0.49–0.90, $P = .02$); (3) patients with a single chest tube had a shorter hospitalization (95% CI: 0.12–0.91, $P = .01$). On the other hand, the results of redrainage rate and postoperative complications showed no significant differences between a single and 2 chest drains.[16]

These data demonstrate that a single chest tube is as effective as 2 drains in achieving air and fluid drainage from the chest cavity after pulmonary resection, and that it is more effective than 2 tubes in terms of postoperative pain, drain duration, and overall hospitalization. Therefore, for these reasons, the authors recommend the use of a single chest tube following an uncomplicated lobectomy.

Furthermore, Gómez-Caro and colleagues[17] suggested the use of a single chest drain following more invasive surgery: in fact, they report no postoperative complications and an adequate overall pleural cavity drainage following 5 chest wall resections and 1 combined lung + diaphragm resection, and in bronchial/arterial sleeve resections.[17]

The authors of this article also adopted a single tube placement after extended resections (14 "en bloc" chest wall + lung resection) (**Fig. 4**) without significant differences in terms of chest tube drainage and duration, but with a meaningful reduction of postoperative pain (Filosso PL, unpublished data, 2015). The authors currently place a single chest tube after an anatomic lung resection (see **Fig. 3**), with the exception of the upper bilobectomy, in which they prefer to place 2 drains, since they observed some cases of inadequate lung re-expansion and persistent air leak that required redrainage. In such cases, the authors used a small-bore chest tube (UNICO; Redax, Poggio Rusco, Italy) placed anteriorly in the II/III intercostal space, to improve the lung re-expansion (**Fig. 5**).

Commonly, large-bore chest drains (24 Fr–32 Fr) are the ones used after pulmonary resections. However, some investigators[18,19] suggested the use of small-bore drains, along with small spiral silicone tubes (Blake tubes) (**Fig. 6**) following lung resections. The major advantages of the latter are a

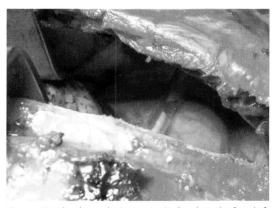

Fig. 4. Single chest drain posteriorly placed after left upper lobectomy and rib resections.

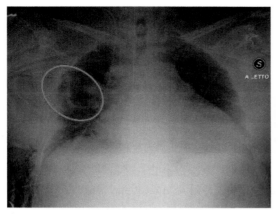

Fig. 5. Postoperative day 2 chest radiograph after right upper bilobectomy: the patient experienced inadequate lung re-expansion, persistent air leak, and subcutaneous emphysema. A small-bore 12-Fr drain (UNICO; *red circle*) was successfully placed and the lung re-expanded after 3 days.

more immediate and effective fluid flow and output due to the long and continuous groove, which theoretically prevents a possible blockage caused by dense fluids or blood. Such drains have been routinely used after breast or thyroid surgery. Suction is however always required in spiral tubes to achieve a fluid drainage comparable to the conventional ones. Moreover, if air leak is present, air evacuation tends to be insufficient even during suction.[20] In the recently published clinical experiences, one[21] or two[22] spiral drains demonstrated to be as effective as traditional tubes for the evacuation of pleural fluid and air after pulmonary resections, being also less painful than the large-bore ones.

Very recently, the authors had the opportunity to test a new device (Smart Drain Coaxial, REDAX Poggiorusco, Italy) that combines the characteristics of these 2 drains: the presence of a continuous groove tube along with external holes, which permit an easier and more effective air output than the traditional spiral system. The preliminary clinical experience (unpublished data) refers to 8 patients submitted to an uncomplicated lobectomy in which a single Smart Drain Coaxial was placed; the results, in terms of fluid and air output, were comparable to the conventional drains.

Because issues such as how much suction or suction versus no suction to apply to the drain are addressed in other specific articles of this issue, the maximum daily amount of fluid output to safely remove the chest tube will not be discussed here.

The recent European Society of Thoracic Surgeons, American Association of Thoracic Surgeons, Society of Thoracic Surgeons, and General Thoracic Surgical Club guidelines for the pleural space management[23] stated that the development of symptomatic pleural effusions, which may require redrainage or other interventional procedures within a month after the chest tube removal, could be regarded as reasonably related to the thoracic surgery and chest drain management. Therefore, this should be regarded as a postoperative complication end point for future studies related to the management of chest drains.

In conclusion, even if several general thoracic surgery textbooks currently recommend the use of 2 chest drains after lobectomy, it has been recently reported in the literature that similar results in terms of air and fluid output drainage may be achieved with the use of a single chest tube. Furthermore, the use of a single chest drain has been demonstrated to be more effective than 2 in reducing postoperative pain, in facilitating patients to adhere to postoperative physiotherapy, and in decreasing the risk of possible respiratory complications. Moreover, the hospitalization and its related costs are reduced with

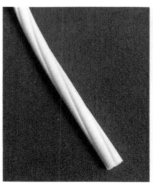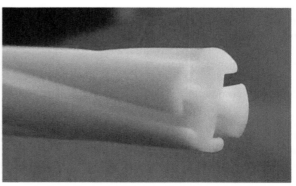

Fig. 6. An example of silicon spiral chest drain the authors are currently using. (*Courtesy of* Redax, Poggio Rusco, Italy; with permission.)

the adoption of a single chest drain, because it is usually removed sooner. Spiral drains have been tested in recent clinical experience, and the results seem to be comparable to conventional drains. Further randomized trials are needed before concluding that a single chest tube should be considered the standard after an uncomplicated lobectomy.

REFERENCES

1. Miserocchi G, Beretta E, Rivolta I. Respiratory mechanics and fluid dynamics after lung resection surgery. Thorac Surg Clin 2010;20:345–57.
2. Albertine KH, Wiener-Kronish JP, Roos PJ, et al. Structure, blood supply, and lymphatic vessels of the sheep's visceral pleura. Am J Anat 1982;165:277–94.
3. Mariassy AT, Wheeldon EB. The pleura: a combined light microscopic, scanning, and transmission electron microscopic study in the sheep. I. Normal pleura. Exp Lung Res 1983;4:293–314.
4. Miserocchi G. Physiology and pathophysiology of pleural fluid turnover. Eur Respir J 1997;10:219–25.
5. Miserocchi G, Negrini D, Gonano C. Parenchymal stress affects interstitial and pleural pressures in situ lung. J Appl Physiol (1985) 1991;71:1967–72.
6. Miserocchi G, Negrini D, Passi A, et al. Development of lung edema: interstitial fluid dynamics and molecular structure. News Physiol Sci 2001;16:66–71.
7. Negrini D, Passi A, Moriondo A. The role of proteoglycans in pulmonary edema development. Intensive Care Med 2008;34:610–8.
8. Lai-Fook SJ. Mechanics of the pleural space: fundamental concepts. Lung 1987;165:249–67.
9. Haber R, Grotberg JB, Glucksberg MR, et al. Steady-state pleural fluid flow and pressure and the effects of lung buoyancy. J Biomech Eng 2001;123:485–92.
10. Fell SC, DeCamp MM. Technical aspects of lobectomy. In: Shields TW, LoCicero J III, Reed CE, et al, editors. General thoracic surgery. Philadelphia: Lippincott Williams & Wilkins; 2009. p. 421–44.
11. Khan IH, Vaughan R. A national survey of thoracic surgical practice in the UK. Int J Clin Pract 1999;53:252–6.
12. Mattioli S, Berrisford RG, Lugaresi ML, et al. Survey on chest drainage systems adopted in Europe. Interact Cardiovasc Thorac Surg 2008;7:1155–9.
13. Filosso PL, Sandri A, Felletti G, et al. Preliminary results of a new small-bore percutaneous pleural catheter used for treatment of malignant pleural effusions in ECOG PS 3-4 patients. Eur J Surg Oncol 2011;37:1093–8.
14. Alex J, Ansari J, Bahalkar P, et al. Comparison of the immediate postoperative outcome of using the conventional two drains versus a single drain after lobectomy. Ann Thorac Surg 2003;76:1046–9.
15. Tanaka M, Sagawa M, Usuda K, et al. Postoperative drainage with one chest tube is appropriate for pulmonary lobectomy: a randomized trial. Tohoku J Exp Med 2014;232:55–61.
16. Zhou D, Deng XF, Liu QX, et al. Single chest tube drainage is superior to double chest tube drainage after lobectomy: a meta-analysis. J Cardiothorac Surg 2016;11:88.
17. Gómez-Caro A, Roca MJ, Torres J, et al. Successful use of a single chest drain postlobectomy instead of two classical drains: a randomized study. Eur J Cardiothorac Surg 2006;29:562–6.
18. Pawelczyk K, Marciniak M, Kacprzak G, et al. One or two drains after lobectomy? A comparison of both methods in the immediate postoperative period. Thorac Cardiovasc Surg 2007;55:313–6.
19. Okur E, Baysungur V, Tezel C, et al. Comparison of the single or double chest tube applications after pulmonary lobectomies. Eur J Cardiothorac Surg 2009;35:32–5.
20. Sakakura N, Fukui T, Mori S, et al. Fluid drainage and air evacuation characteristics of Blake and conventional drains used after pulmonary resection. Ann Thorac Surg 2009;87:1539–45.
21. Niinami H, Tabata M, Takeuchi Y, et al. Experimental assessment of the drainage capacity of small silastic chest drains. Asian Cardiovasc Thorac Ann 2006;14:223–6.
22. Terzi A, Feil B, Bonadiman C, et al. The use of flexible spiral drains after non-cardiac thoracic surgery. A clinical study. Eur J Cardiothorac Surg 2005;27:134–7.
23. Brunelli A, Beretta E, Cassivi SD, et al. Consensus definitions to promote an evidence-based approach to management of the pleural space. A collaborative proposal by ESTS, AATS, STS, and GTSC. Eur J Cardiothorac Surg 2011;40:291–7.

Thoracic Trauma
Which Chest Tube When and Where?

Tamas F. Molnar, MD, PhD, DSc, FETS[a,b],*

KEYWORDS

- Chest trauma • Traumatic hemo/pneumothorax • Emergency surgery • Mass casualty • Triage

KEY POINTS

- Penetrating and blunt trauma (with or without rib fracture) needs different tactics according to mechanism of injury.
- Selective conservativism and drainage surmounted pleural space control are dominating optimally invasive chest trauma management.
- Massive bleeding and/or trapped intrapleural air causing high intrathoracic pressure are the 2 main catastrophic but potentially survivable events, in which decompression by a drain offers a simple and efficient solution in 90% to 95% of all cases.
- Many failed but still existing dogmas and misunderstandings surrounding hemo/pneumothorax, ill interpretation of "horror vacui pleurae," prevents a more proactive surgical attitude toward this method among nonthoracic surgeons and allied specialists.
- Experience-based convictions and received wisdom prevails as only a limited number of statistically controlled evidence exists.

INTRODUCTION

Life is really simple, but we insist on making it complicated (Confucius).

Only a few life-threatening conditions in trauma surgery are potentially manageable by a simple and straightforward intervention with a good chance of success. Chest drainage, the release of murderously high intrapleural pressure caused by accumulated and trapped blood (hemothorax) and/or air (pneumothorax) is just that sort of minor surgery offering a dramatic effect. In spite of the uncomplicated clinical picture of tension hemo/pneumothorax, the uncomplicated decision making and the simplicity of the procedure, missed/failed pleural decompression might be responsible for up to 33% of the preventable fatalities typically in combat and in a lesser but increasing degree in civilian environments.[1,2] Changing urban criminal/terrorist action injury profiles[3,4] and challenges of mass casualty care and disaster medical management equally warrant a more focused analysis of the seemingly simple and frequently neglected intervention of chest drainage. The rapid clinical decline caused by the compression of the underlying lung and mediastinum with profuse bleeding highlights the importance of the prehospital care and/or first medical responder treatment of these patients. However, chest injury is only an element of a complex severe clinical scenario in a good number of serious cases. Approximately 60% of multi/polytrauma patients suffer chest trauma

Disclosure Statement: The author has nothing to disclose.
[a] Department of Operational Medicine, Faculty of Medicine, University of Pécs, H7622 Pécs, Szigeti út 12, Hungary; [b] Thoracic Surgery Unit, Department of Surgery, Aladar Petz Teaching Hospital, H9032 Győr, Vasvari Pál utca 2-4, Hungary
* H.7625 Magaslati u 35 II.8, Pécs, Hungary.
E-mail address: tfmolnar@gmail.com

among other injuries.[5] Thoracic injury is responsible for the death in 1 of 4 or 5 fatalities. Quick and efficient control of the pleural space by drainage plays a double role in the context of current resuscitation concept (CBABC) at least in military trauma paradigm[6] by removing intrapleural blood (Catastrophic Bleeding) and relieving compromised breathing (B) at the same time. The evidence-based scientific approach of the state of art in hemo/pneumothorax is not a trouble-free zone due to a practically complete lack of externally controlled data. The literature is rich in audit-style retrospective reports in which the results with chest drainage for trauma cases are described and discussed.[7,8] However, as usual, the devil lurks in the particulars. What insertion technique using what type and size of drain, followed by which tactics of suction treatment; these questions are considered scientifically irrelevant, too down-to-earth details, and therefore remain unreported. Chest drainage is the Cinderella in the shadow of heroic surgeries of major torso trauma. Autoreflective reports present the success of their own method, which is excellent. Publications are ruled by an extremely high success rate: 90% to 95% of all penetrating chest wound cases are treated exclusively by intercostal chest drains (ICDs).[9,10] In fact, no more than 18% to 22% of all injuries involving the thorax require chest drainage for pneumo/hemothorax and approximately 1 in 10 to 14 initially drained patients has to undergo major thoracic surgery.[5] Sixty percent to 75% of all chest drainages are performed for penetrating injuries. Distribution of hemothorax and pneumothorax as indications are roughly equal, whereas the last third of the group consists of the combined, that is, hemopneumothorax cases.[10]

Acute trauma–related pleural space management by chest drains is a field of received wisdom, in which the basic principles are neither questioned nor investigated in full depth. The present article is the result of an attempt of a structured review of the problems and of the annotated listing of the orthodox solutions rather than an analysis of nonexistent evidence.

A distillate of personal experience of 30 years filtered through the recent literature on chest drainage in trauma is presented. Other articles in this issue should be consulted especially where retained hemothorax and primary thoracic empyema[11] are concerned. Chest trauma is discussed "per se," as an acute event; therefore, the role of chest drainage in treatment of sequelae and consequences of thoracic injuries is not discussed here.

SURGICAL TECHNIQUE

Rudyard Kipling delineated the framework of the discussion of chest drainage technicalities in trauma. "I keep six honest serving-men. They taught me all I knew. Their names are What and Why and When and How and Where and Who."[12] The only modification required is the rearrangement of the names into a when-why-where-what-how-who sequence, as art of surgery has a different logic from poetry.

When

One of the beauties of chest drainage in thoracic trauma is that the decision-making process does not contain a lot of steps: in extremis no imaging is needed at all before the procedure. Vast clinical experience teaches that physical examination has an utmost importance here.[7,9,13]

Chest drainage should be performed immediately whenever the serious suspicion of tension pneumothorax or massive hemothorax[5,14] is aroused based on clinical signs in a patient who has shortness of breath or is simply hypoxic. The clinical signs are as follows: decreased deflection on one side of the chest cage, no or minimal breathing sounds are audible on the affected side, drumlike sounds with percussion in case of pneumothorax and dullness for hemothorax, and the trachea palpated in the sternal notch is pressed to the opposite side. Pulse oximetry can provide adjunctive informations, just like extended focused assessment sonography in trauma (e-FAST). Level 2 recommendation supports the use of e-FAST in chest trauma.[15] Chest radiograph (CXR), the oldest imaging method of diagnosing pneumo/hemothorax has a reported disappointing sensitivity of less than 50%.[16] Excluding occult and minimal (<10%) pneumothorax and if only significant pneumothoraces are counted, then this value is significantly higher. Computed tomography (CT) has a near 100% sensitivity, but it is far from being the optimal diagnostic tool in unstable patients. e-FAST has a sensitivity of 77% for pneumothorax with a negative predictive factor just below 100%.[17]

Why

Mechanism of injury: that is, blunt versus penetrating trauma, dictates different surgical decision making. Generally speaking, penetrating injuries entering the pleural space nearly always call for a chest drain, with 2 exceptions. On one hand, there are those penetrating, usually impaled injuries, that are obvious straightforward thoracotomy cases (see later in this article) without prior drainage, whereas on the other hand, the symptom-free patients with a stab wound whose pneumothorax is smaller than 2 cm, also can wait.[18] There are opinions for a (nearly) immediate discharge of asymptomatic penetrating trauma cases, with negative CXR,[13] whereas others are a little bit more cautious. Physiologic parameters and imaging are steering the decisions less aggressively in cases of blunt thoracic injuries usually complicated by rib/sternum fracture.[5,14]

Drainage of the pleural space has to have definitive aims, but surgical correction of a radiologic picture is not one of them. Pneumothorax less than 10% or 2 cm and symptomless does not require a chest drain.[18] However, these patients need to be monitored for at least 24 hours.[19] It is worth remembering that for more than 60 years, pneumothorax was induced artificially as a sole treatment in the hope of cure of tuberculosis; so a limited amount of intrapleural air does not cause any harm. The military surgical experience during World War I saw benefit of air replacement of the tapped hemothorax,[20] a common procedure for lung tuberculosis in the age. What is obvious in contemporary practice is that preinjury inherent reserves of the ventilatory capacities are decisive in the outcome.

Hemothorax is a different case, in which amount of original volume and tendency commands a different approach.[14,21] Any hemothorax responsible for ventilatory compromise needs to be drained immediately.

An open pneumothorax (sucking chest wound), in which the pleural space is in a definite and permanent continuation with the surrounding atmospheric environment (permanent hole, destroyed/missing full-depth chest wall, sucking chest wound) needs a secure cover and a drain. Alternatively, dressings/covers with a built-in 1-way valve are available (SAM [Vented; SAM Medical Products, The Netherlands, The Hague], HALO [Halo VENT Chest Seal; Halo Automotive, USA], Ashermann Chest Seal [Teleflex Medical, Coventry, CT, USA], Bolin [H&H Medical Corporation, Williamsburg, VA, USA], and Russell Chest Seal [Prometheus Medical Ltd, Hope Under Dinmore, Herefordshire, UK] and other models based on slightly different concepts). No independent comparative study is available on their performance in the clinical setting.[22]

Where

The side of pneumothorax/hemothorax should be marked before the procedure, the CXR/CT/Chest ultrasound consulted and communicated to the staff, and finally checked again. There is a general

agreement on the optimal location of the chest drainage,[23] a rare exception, as so many divergent opinions coexist on this topic. The patient is lying in a mild head-up position (anti-Trendelenburg or Fowler position) with the affected side up. The midaxillary or the anterior axillary line offers an ideally thin layer of the chest wall muscles and the fifth or sixth intercostal spaces (between the fifth and sixth or sixth and seventh ribs, respectively) are mentioned more frequently.[24,25] Go lower in this safe triangle and you might find your tube in the abdomen or just too close to the diaphragm; or go higher and the subpulmonary region of the pleural space will be left without effective evacuation. Chest tubes do not need to be directed posteriorly,[26] but an upward position is advantageous. The above site recommendation is true in the relatively rare cases of thoracic monotrauma. The advice loses its relevance when either a polytrauma patient is treated by a team or prehospital resuscitation is performed.[27] Where a multitrauma or polytrauma patient in a supine position is considered, and the primary survey is under way, there are 2 choices of drain sites. One might follow the axillary route, detailed previously, or an anterior approach in which the second or third intercostal space is entered. The former might be somewhat uncomfortable for the surgeon from an ergonomic point of view, whereas the latter is complicated by the stout pectoral muscle mass.

No other evidence than massive expert opinion and common sense support the practice.

What

The size of tube and of hemothorax to be evacuated are equally important determinants.[5,28] The material of the drain has an utmost importance, as it must be flexible and resilient but should resist the compression in the intercostal tunnel and intrapleural kinking. Silicon, an ideal component for soft abdominal drains, is unsuitable above the diaphragm. Unrevealed occluded chest drains are deceiving to the surgeon, suggesting patency falsely. The tubes must be multiholed and should be marked for CXRs. As far as size is concerned, there is a general agreement on the recommendation of between 28 and 30-French gauge (Ch) for an average adult and larger for larger body and/or massive hemothorax. A smaller diameter might work in selected cases, pigtail is not excluded,[29] and a more flexible approach is permitted where pure pneumothorax is concerned.[30]

How

Obtain written consent of the patient if applicable and available and document if not. Explain the procedure to the patient and share your plans with the staff. Double-check the side. Surgical technique consists of 4 basic steps: (1) skin incision and tunneling, (2) entering the chest cavity and introducing the drain, (3) fixing the tube, and (4) finally connecting it to the suction with detailed instructions on how to manage the system.

The skin incision should allow the maneuvering of the tube through the chest wall and into the pleural space. The size of the drain defines the length of the incision in less than an inch (1.5–2.0 cm). There are 3 methods of passing the tube into the desired place and position. First, the oldest and nowadays old-fashioned way of pleural detention is using a trocar and introducing the drain through it. The second option is the application of some derivative of the mandrin, another French medical word, which is an inverted, "inside-out" trocar. The chest drain is pulled over a guiding rod or thin stylet in its full length. There is an endless list of different ready-made single-use chest drain kits on the market based on the same principle: introducing the rod-tube complex and then remove the rigid inner part. All models share the same disadvantage: as the tip of the complex enters the pleural space, no one knows exactly where it will end. There is no intrathoracic organ that this skewer, ideal for an open-air shashlik roasting party, did not perforate, according to collected data and individual case reports.[31–33] The method is recommendable only for complete and total traumatic pneumothorax and/or massive hemothorax. Industrial interference on the medical device market and surgical idleness are responsible for the overpermeation of the technology.

Blunt dissection of the subcutaneous tissue, then the intercostal layer using a Pean/Roberts forceps in a step-by-step manner, provides the safest approach to the pleural space. The index finger may complete the innermost 1 to 2 mm of the tunnel and enter the chest cavity. As the tip of the drain safely enters the pleural space, use the Pean/Roberts forceps to steer it into the direction of the apical region of the chest cage. Attention must be paid so that the last side-hole is well within the pleural cavity, otherwise it tends to slip out, causing surgical emphysema.

There are no comparative studies with regard to the relative values of the 3 different techniques. The authors' nonevidenced subjective but educated guess is that thoracic surgeons and many trauma specialists prefer the last method, whereas nonsurgical specialists, such as emergency doctors, intensive therapists, and junior staff, prefer the mandrin method.

Chest drainage is a surgical intervention, whatever small and/or quick procedure it should be.

Proper indication, safe technique, and close control after care are 3 equally important pillars of success. Preparations include consent (bypassable only in unconscious patients), local anesthesia, and systemic pain control during and after intervention. Antibiotics are a question of debate, as hard evidence that is based on observational rather than randomized studies is inconsistent. A pooled analysis of 1234 patients revealed that antibiotic prophylaxis resulted in an almost 3 times lower risk of empyema than those who did not receive antibiotic treatment. The infection rate was reduced impressively in the subgroup of penetrating chest injuries. Blunt trauma subgroup did not benefit from antibiotic prophylaxis.[34] There seems to be an agreement on the need of a single-dose prophylactic antibiotic, in spite of growing concerns of antibiotic abuse and subsequent multidrug resistance. Common sense also dictates a self-restraining policy in pneumothorax cases, whereas penetrating chest injuries demand antibiotic prophylaxis.[35] Skin disinfection and pain control, frequently undervalued, should be integral parts of proper drainage.[36]

The ways of securing the tube to the skin, preventing dislodgement, surgical emphysema, and falling out are numerous. The simplest way is to use 2 string of ties: one for anchorage and one for closing the wound when the tube is removed. Common sense dictates using stranded cord (0 or stronger), as it is less slippery than coated or monofilament surgical thread. Many of us prefer 2-in-1 solutions: in which the thread is coiled around the tube in multiple rounds and is spun in reverse when the tube is removed and tied as a simple wound closure. Every thoracic surgeon has developed his or her own method, as has the present author (**Fig. 1**). The traditional "Roman sandal" method with alpha-cross-wires[37] seems to be less than ideal.[38] The method has its modifications[39] but independent comparison results are still awaited. Insufficient securing of the tube takes its revenge not only in slipping out, but in surgical emphysema, as well.[40]

Who

Chest drainage as an emergency procedure should be performed by any manual specialists. This is a basic competence, the same as cricothyrotomy or application of a tourniquet bandage in profuse bleeding of an extremity. The local rules may vary from country to country, usually delegating the procedure to emergency medical doctors in a prehospital trauma setting. It might be said, that in an in-hospital emergency department setting, a first-come, first-serve rule is preferable

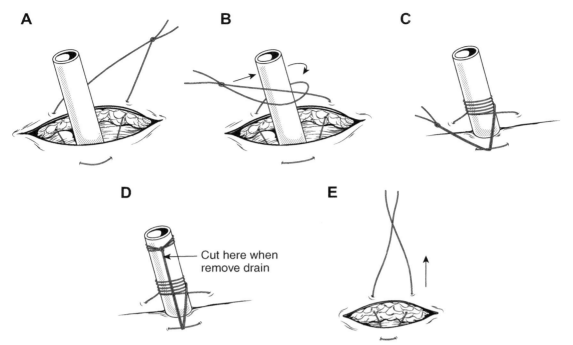

Fig. 1. Two in 1: how to fix the drain securely with a 2-in-1 stitch, which will close the wound at removal. (*A–C*) Steps of securing the drain to the skin. (*D, E*) Steps to be taken at removal of the drain.

to waiting until a thoracic surgeon shows up. As is expected, seniority helps: complication rate, even security of fixing ties, are closely related with experience.[32,33,38] However, this fact should not limit junior staff activity. There is no such thing as too much training in the concept and exercise of chest drainage.

Again, no reliable published prospective data are available on this paragraph.

PREOPERATIVE PLANNING

Running against time: this is a decisive feature of primary treatment for chest trauma. The very first step of planning is establishing a diagnosis of thoracic injury and confirming need of relieving an acute pleural space–occupying progressive condition. Mechanism of injury (eg, weapon, circumstances of road traffic accident) offers important clues for surgical decision making. Paramedic and emergency medical service reports (written and/or oral) and pressure marks on the skin are helpful. Scars of previous chest surgeries (ie, thoracotomy, sternotomy) should warn the surgeon to expect extensive intrathoracic adhesions. Previous pleural inflammations also might pose a trap during insertion of the tube.

Second to the prior physical examinations (inspection, feeling, percussion, auscultation), basic imaging is considered. The gross pathologies

requiring immediate chest drainage are obvious even on rudimentary radiological means. CXR is losing territory to CT. Emergency ultrasound and e-FAST support a decision when physical examination does not provide a clear yes/no answer for drainage. Chest CT helps, but is rarely needed for the decision on emergency draining of the thorax. When drainage is performed, it is a primary diagnostic procedure with a 90% to 95% chance that it is therapeutic as well, especially if the injury involves the periphery of the thoracic domain.

A patient with chest injury with traumatic arrest without cardiac output should need immediate decompression: bilateral drainage to exclude tension pneumothorax. The expected "diagnosis ex juvantibus" does not allow time to wait for imaging studies. A patient with penetrating chest trauma in shock and with profound hypoxemia also needs to be drained in an attempt at restoring physiologic intrapleural environment.

Chest drainage is equal or superior to video-assisted thoracoscopic surgery (VATS) exploration in acute injury in terms of providing vital information: is there a need for immediate thoracotomy to identify the source of bleeding and control? Drainage can be performed without the risks and time, staff consumption of general anesthesia, and single lung ventilation of a completely unknown patient. VATS or minimally invasive open thoracic surgery (MAOTS) is ideal for the stabilized patient, in an elective surgery setting, providing one has the anesthesia backup, proper experience, and hospital budget. In most acute trauma cases, no time is left for delicate minimally invasive procedures. Profuse bleeding blinds the camera, and if not, then there was no need for VATS.

IMMEDIATE POSTPROCEDURAL CARE

The final outcome is strongly dependent on postoperative care, which begins with the connection of the chest drain to the adjacent systems. Written instructions for the staff (suction force, CXR schedules) help in avoiding communication breakdown, especially as drained chest cases are relatively rare in trauma wards/bays. Suction systems irrespective of their type (1-way valve, Heimlich or Bülau type, passive or active suction) are extensions of the pleural space. Force of suction in case of active suction is a question of local hospital policy. The numbers are variable between 10 and 50 cm H_2O and every thoracic and trauma consultant has his or her watertight reason for her or his own particular practice. Suction regulators and drainage systems are discussed elsewhere in this issue. It must be stated here that the simplest system is better for the outcome. There are computer-controlled mobile active suction devices available. Although their affordability and cost-benefit ratios are questionable, their advantage of freeing the patient from his or her bed is out of question. The junior staff and the nurses should understand the principle of suction applied, be familiar with the system used, and troubleshooting must be straightforward. This is extremely important in emergency ward/trauma departments where suction systems are not part of the daily routine, as they are in a general thoracic surgical unit/department. Regular control of the patency of the system, volume, and quality (hematocrit!) of evacuated fluid is also mandatory. Physical status of the chest should be checked by the junior staff at least twice a day. Intervals of CXR control are questions of debate, in which patient safety, diagnostic benefit, and the shadow of a litigation case out of the blue are struggling with each other. In the absence of any reliable guideline, the author's practice is presented here. If anything happens (drain repositioned, removed, changed, suction tactics modified, patient's condition deteriorated, serious complaints aroused) an erect position CXR is requested (preferably bedside) to check the situation and document. Documentation of all details is mandatory, and this is in the best interest of the staff and the patient.

The chest tube is removable when no further air escape is detected. The swinging fluid in the connecting tube is a sign of cessation of active air leakage from the pleural surface. Being that 200 to 300 mL/24-hour fluid evacuation is the universally accepted threshold in case of malignant pleural effusion, the same value also may orient the surgeon in case of chest trauma. All in all, the recommendations for patients with chest trauma drainage do not differ significantly from the tasks to be fulfilled in general thoracic surgical cases. Pain control needs increased attention, even though the patient population is younger, frequently free of underlying lung diseases, and expectations are good, especially if the polytrauma sufferers are excluded.

Clinical Results in the Literature

The very nature of chest trauma and the heterogeneity of the patient pool and causes explains the lack of publications with a high degree of evidence. Declarations are ruling the field rather than crystallized consensus. The reported results are contradictory; the meta-analyses are suffering from all sorts of bias. Chest drainage in thoracic trauma is not a topic at the present time and is unlikely that it get over the top where randomized trial overwrite the ruling practice. Approximately 150 years of collective memories and experience provide the backbone of our received wisdom. The reader is referred to the reference list to find the available sources. However, this shortcoming should not disappoint, but motivate the new generation of trauma, chest, and general surgeons and emergency doctors to conduct prospective, ideally multicenter, and wherever possible, randomized trials on the questions exposed or not covered here.

An alibi comparison of uncomparable data would not serve the noble aim of a review on the erritory of chest drainage in thoracic trauma. References to complication and conversion rates are useful only at the population level, and have no relevance for the individual case. They can be used for quality control and litigation/malpractice lawsuits, but tell nothing to the surgeon in the middle of the night standing in a trauma bay.

Alternatives to Chest Drainage

Special circumstances and shortcomings in trained hands dictate need for alternatives to chest drainage in certain situations and cases. Limitations in competence and extremely dangerous/hostile (care under fire) and contaminated environments favor needle decompression, preferred by the military.[27] In spite of suboptimal results (mainly for too thick chest wall musculature), it has its own merit. Intrapleural relieving procedures performed by drainage are considered universally beyond combat medic/civilian paramedic–level competences.

Too high frequency of insufficient on-site chest drainage in prehospital care led to the concept of emergency thoracostomy in ventilated patients.[41] More data are awaited; however, it is unclear why the axillary approach is preferred instead of the more obvious anterior chest wall limited size opening. It is quite convincing that creating an escape route for trapped air/fluid in a closed space, while oxygenation is maintained artificially is preferable to a drain with dubious patency.

When Not to Attempt to Drain the Chest at All (Exclusion Criteria)

There are scenarios when chest drainage for thoracic trauma is only a waste of time. Extensively destroyed chest wall/lung or impaled objects might call for immediate open surgery.[42] Penetrating wounds, either from a projectile or stabbing, in the projection of the heart anteriorly or posteriorly, demand surgical exploration of the chest. A cardiothoracic surgeon with capacity of an immediate intervention at any time and ruling all necessity facilities might decide otherwise (focused diagnostics, special monitoring devices) but generally this is not the case. As a rule, suspicion of heart/great vessel injury is amenable to immediate surgical intervention. An unnecessary exploration is the lesser evil and the judgment is always "a posteriori." A thoracic exploration is a highly survivable procedure, whereas a missed penetrating heart or major vascular injury is definitely not.

When to Convert Chest Drainage to Thoracotomy

There is an ongoing wrestling with the numbers of milliliters where the drainage/thoracotomy threshold is concerned. As usual, it is a multifaceted, multifactorial question to answer. The key players are volume, time of evacuation, age, physiologic reserves, circumstances, and other factors are to be considered. Thoracotomy has its own inherent mortality of 0.25% to 0.5%. More than 1500 mL loss of blood at once or 300 mL per hour for more than 4 hours are the universally accepted values as indications for thoracotomy.[5] Unfortunately, systemic hemostatics (eg, factor VII, tranexamic acid) are usually not considered as adjunct to the treatment. One should keep in mind during transfusion, that what the patient is losing and might need to be replaced is fresh full blood.

POTENTIAL COMPLICATIONS/MANAGEMENT

No intervention is without risks and chest drainage in trauma, typically under stress of time, multitasking, and relative individuality of the challenges is not an exception. It is not uncommon that problem solving becomes the problem itself. Scapegoating does not help: one never can forget that it is the trauma itself that is the origo of complications; surgical mistakes only follow. In an age in which the pseudo culture of complaints and Damocles' sword of litigation hangs above us, this basic truth is too frequently forgotten. It is a misconception to suppose that all complications are avoidable. Saying that, one has to emphasize, that it does not exempt us from paying the utmost attention and concentration during chest drainage and beyond in thoracic injury.

All imaginable and even unimaginable types of complications of drains in chest trauma, not a few with fatal outcomes, are described and many more never saw paper. These procedures are performed in a rush against time in a desperate situation in a hope of stopping the complete fall of the dominoes. A varying number and severity of complications can be avoided or at least reduced with proper protocols and training, but a complete preemption is a logical impossibility. It is the trauma that kills at the end and not the attending surgeon/emergency doctor.

As ICD is a lifesaving procedure in a great number of cases, the risks cannot be balanced against the benefits if the slightest suspicion for the need for ICD would arise. The only mistake is the one that ICD (or alternatives: ie, needle decompression, decompressive thoracostomy in an intubated patient) was not performed when it was needed. A missed tension pneumothorax or massive hemothorax are nonforgiving killers. The complication rate varies between 2% and 10%.[32,33] Most complications are minor ones, like kinking or displacement, slipping out, or surgical emphysema. Only 2% to 3% of all chest drain mistakes result in serious collateral damage, like perforation, with a mortality of 20% to 25%.[32]

Immediate Complications

Vascular

The process of insertion of the tube might cause further bleeding by vessel injury. Intercostal artery and/or vein (60%–75% of all serious complications) can suffer tangential rupture. Injury of the subclavian artery, either by the tip of the inserting rod or the tube itself, is rare: 5% to 7% of all major perforations. Any other intrathoracic vessel can be injured, of course. Minor vascular traumas are self-healing (the drain is tamponading), whereas massive bleeding requires immediate exploration. The author prefers open but muscle-sparing exploration (axillary thoracotomy, minimal access open thoracotomy [MAOT]) to VATS.

Cardiac complications
The heart is involved in 16% of all serious collateral damage incidents.[33] Immediate thoracotomy should be attempted, and mortality is high. Dysrhythmias pose either as immediate or late complications, depending on the onset of the drain-caused myocardial irritation. Solution: withdrawing the tube or changing the site of the drain.

Lung parenchyma
In 10% to 12% of all serious injuries, collateral damage involves pulmonary parenchyma. The author's impression is that lung parenchyma is more vulnerable if mandrins are used. Previous adhesions, intrapleural strings can be disrupted, resulting in tears on the lung surface or bleeding (see previously). Bronchopleural, pleurocutaneous fistulas can be produced by prolonged tubes, especially if the drain material is too rigid. On some occasions in which subsequent surgery is needed, tubes are mistakenly reported as being tunneled into the depth of the lung parenchyma. Actually, lung parenchyma tends to embrace the tube, surrounding it and giving the false impression of a deeply penetrated tube into the pulmonary tissue itself. CT images can be misleading in this aspect. Solution: at first, shortening the intrathoracic part of the tube might help. Complete removal of the tube with leaving the drain site open in a thoracostomy fashion is another option. By this time, the adhesions that have developed usually prevent collapse of the lung. Surgical exploration (MAOS, VATS) and closure of the fistula or limited resection of the involved part of the lung might be needed as a last resort.

Other organs
Diaphragm laceration (30% of all major complications), perforation, and consequences of abdominal cavity penetration can result in injury of stomach (20%), colon (2%–3%), spleen (10%–30%), or liver (5%–7%). Esophagus (3%–5%) and kidney (1%) are rarely involved. Solution: exploration of the abdomen either laparoscopically or via open access. Solving the life-threatening chest condition has a priority, and the abdominal phase follows only in a stabilized patient.[33] Two of 3 perforations require exploration and surgical correction (laparoscopy, laparotomy, VATS, MAOT, open thoracotomy).

Pleural shock
Vagal reflex can produce cardiac arrest in extremely rare occasions. Solution: resuscitation, intensive care.

Expansion edema
The pathology described after relieving of long-standing pneumothorax or pleural fluid accumulation is, theoretically speaking, a possibility after trauma, also. However, the danger posed by the intrapleural compression far exceeds the distant dangers of a too-quick lung expansion; therefore, no staged decompression is advised in the chest trauma setting.

Drainage on the wrong side
This is the only complication that must be absolutely avoided. This is a rare, but serious mistake, originating only in negligence.

Complications in the Early Phase

Surgical emphysema (subcutaneous emphysema)
Collected air in the subcutaneous region in the vicinity of the tube or more extensively in the upper torso and head (Michelin-tire figure) is the sign of a blocked tube and a still-active air escape from the pleural surface. Malposition of the Heimlich valve, blocking air escape, causing massive pneumothorax and surgical emphysema is extremely rare.[43] Always consider gas-producing bacteria also, but in most cases the chest tube is blocked usually by a clot. Either the patient lies on it, or a tube kinking or dislocation occurs, the drain slips out a bit and the last side-hole (most distal from the tip) crawls into the muscle layers of the chest wall. Ask the nurse, if she or he clamped the tube for a while. Solution: control the patency of the tube (clot) and put the patient on high-value suction. Aiming at quick symptomatic relief, the skin might be incised or a small-caliber subcutaneous short-tube insertion can speed up the resolution. Explanation and reassurance to the patient, relatives, their lawyers, and the nursing staff on the harmless nature of the condition are essential.

Sudden onset of severe pain, shortness of breath
Listen to the lung, check pulse oximeter. Reduce the power of suction and give analgesia. If there is no relief in 30 to 60 minutes, consider changing (withdrawing) the drain a bit.

Content of collection bottle
Sudden change of volume, appearance of fluid in the collection bottles: that is, chyle, gastric/esophageal contents indicates late onset of viscus

perforation. Following a fast-track investigation, identify and treat the complication.

Late Complications

Pleural fistulas with prolonged air escape can originate in the original injury itself (inward tip of fractured rib) or rather commonly in a longstanding, irritating tip of tube.

Thoracic, empyema usually in stage II and III is the most commonly reported postdrainage complication. Paradoxically enough, undrained, retained clotted blood is made responsible for another, non unsignificant portions of secondary (posttraumatic) thoracic empyemas. Posttraumatic empyema developing after drainage is attributed quite unanimously to the procedure rather than a complication of insufficient evacuation or even pneumonia due to suboptimal aftercare (lack of incentive spirometry, inhalation, patient position, extended bed rest). Reality is more complex: usually a combination of the 3 is responsible for the adverse outcome. The condition, if it develops, is better treated by a dedicated thoracic surgical unit/department in an "a frois" phase. Empyema thoracis is a manageable condition with good chances, whereas a tension pneumothorax or a massive intrapleural bleeding kills.

Intercostal/drain site pain is a nuisance for the patient and doctor alike, healed by time in a good number of cases. The prognosis is highly unpredictable. Local anesthetics are advised, but success is not guaranteed. Referral to a pain clinic might help.

SPECIAL CONSIDERATIONS

Chest trauma is rarely limited to the well-fed urban populations with high-tech medical facilities at arm stretch and not only is the civilian population involved. Chest drainage offers hope for many who are seriously injured in extreme situations in peace, disasters, and war alike.

Chest Trauma in Multiple Casualty and Mass Casualty Situations

A mass casualty (MASCAL) situation is marked by an acute discrepancy between the actual treating facilities/capacities and the number and the severity of the injuries of those who are in need as the flow of the patients is too high.[3,44] Unsaturated MASCAL or multiple casualty scenarios (typically urban terrorist attacks) are less demanding in this aspect. The rate of chest injuries in these situations varies from event to event, but its high frequency usually as part of multi/polytrauma rather than a thoracic monotrauma is nondisputable. Simple

detention of life-threatening intrapleural pressure relieves not only the individual patient, but the providing system under extreme stress also. Chest drainage is not a panacea, but is a procedure taking no more than 5 minutes that can reclassify a patient from T1 to T2 or T3 triage group. Chest drainage is a cornerstone in the management of torso injuries in damage control surgery.[45] There is a pendulumlike shift in the preferred procedures for chest trauma. From the Korean war (1950–1953) onward, there is a trend to perform too many unnecessary thoracotomies instead of drainage alone at the beginning of the treatment of the victims of armed conflicts. As experiences are collected, and evaluated, chest drainage regains its proper place in the protocols. The progress restarts at the start of the next war,[20] as surgical dogmas are hard to change.

Prophylactic Drainage

There are institutional protocols for inserting preventive chest drains in the case of serial rib fractures (suspected underlying lung injuries) if the need for artificial ventilation is expected: either for emergency surgery (abdominal, skeletal) or for intensive care. The numbers vary, usually from 3 or 4 broken ribs and up, and there are other factors to evaluate also. Flail chest, spatial relation of bone edges, exact location of the fractures (the lower the better), and nontrauma-related condition of the lung (CT image) are also to be considered. No particular recommendation can be given, but the concept is worth considering.

Limited Pneumo/Hemothorax in the Old and Fragile Patients

With the almost endemic antiplatelet therapy, the frequency of hemothorax cases following very minor trauma[46] reaches heights never seen before in the same manner as subdural hematoma cases are accumulating. These patients need extra attention and a more proactive surgical attitude might be considered. The advice is based purely on personal experience, as no reliable data are available as the question seems to be the holy cow of contemporary medicine.

Extemporary Means: Chest Surgery in War and/or Remote, Rural Regions

There are some minor tricks that make chest drainage possible in challenging environments with limited or no access to the blessings of the tools of modern surgery:

a. In a shortage of proper chest drains, industrial rubber tubes (sterilized in hot water) with improvised multilocular side holes can be used with acceptable effect.

b. In a shortage of drainage systems/sucking bottles and prefabricated Heimlich valves, the holed rubber gloves or condoms fixed to the external tip of the tube provide an improvised but safe 1-way valve.

c. von Bülau's bottle can be improvised from simple jars. The patient's drain should be connected to the upper end of an underwater tube. When another Bülau bottle is used, the air-pipe tube (space above the water) connected to a mouth piece and sucked by the patient makes an improvised incentive spirometry tool. The inhaled air should come against pressure controlled by the depth of the tip of the other tube positioned below water level. Length of the underwater part can be adjusted to the capacities of the patient.

SUMMARY

The Hamlethian question in chest trauma is to drain or not to drain. The answer is that drainage is always to be considered, except with an unstable patient injured in the projection of the heart where straightforward surgery should be performed, just like in obviously extensive thoracic destruction. If drainage cannot control bleeding/air escape, then an immediate open surgical approach should follow. Preinterventional investigations should be minimized, as detention has priority. Without strict written and regularly reviewed institutional protocols and continuous training, there is no chance to avoid complications, exposing patients to unnecessary collateral damage and beyond.

REFERENCES

1. Kotwal RS, Montgomery HR, Kotwal BM, et al. Eliminating preventable death on the battlefield. Arch Surg 2011;146(12):1350–8.

2. Mark AC, Wimberger N, Sztajnkrycer MD. Incidence of tension pneumothorax in police officers feloniously killed in the line of duty: a ten-year retrospective analysis. Prehosp Disaster Med 2012;27(1):94–7.

3. Waage S, Poole JC, Thorgersen EB. Rural hospital mass casualty response to a terrorist shooting spree. Br J Surg 2013;100:1198–204.

4. Hu Y, Zheng X, Yuan Y, et al. Comparison of injury epidemiology between the Wenchuan and Lushan Earthquakes, in Sichuan, China. Disaster Med Public Health Prep 2014;8(6):541–7.

5. Broderick SR. Hemothorax. etiology, diagnosis, and management. Thorac Surg Clin 2013;23:89–96.

6. Hodgetts TJ, Mahoney PF, Russell MQ, et al. ABC to CABC: redefining the military trauma paradigm. Emerg Med J 2006;23(10):745–6.

7. Heus C, Mellema JJ, Giannakopoulos GF, et al. Outcome of penetrating chest injuries in an urban level I trauma center in the Netherlands. Eur J Trauma Emerg Surg 2015;2015:1863–9941.

8. Khorsandi M, Skouras C, Prasad S, et al. Major cardiothoracic trauma: eleven-year review of outcomes in the North West of England. Ann R Coll Surg Engl 2015;97(4):298–303.

9. Blyth A. Thoracic trauma. BMJ 2014;348:g1137.

10. Kong VY, Oosthuizen GV, Clarke DL. Selective conservativism in the management of thoracic trauma remains appropriate in the 21st century. Ann R Coll Surg Engl 2015;97(3):224–8.

11. Molnar TF. Current surgical treatment of thoracic empyema in adults. Eur J Cardiothorac Surg 2007;32(3):422–30.

12. Kipling R. The Elephant's Child. Just So Stories. Available at: https://allpoetry.com/I-Keep-Six-Honest-Serving-Men. Accessed September 30, 2016.

13. Seidzadeh GL, Yari A, Mayel M, et al. Observation period for asymptomatic penetrating chest trauma: 1 or 3 h? Eur J Trauma Emerg Surg 2016;2016:1863–9933.

14. Wells BJ, Roberts DJ, Grondin S, et al. To drain or not to drain? Predictors of tube thoracostomy insertion and outcomes associated with drainage of traumatic haemothoraces. Injury 2015;46:1743–8.

15. Mowery NT, Gunter OL, Collier BR, et al. Practice management guidelines for management of hemothorax and occult pneumothorax. J Trauma 2011;70(2):510–8.

16. Wilkerson RG, Stone MB. Sensitivity of bedside ultrasound and supine anteroposterior chest radiographs for the identification of pneumothorax after blunt trauma. Acad Emerg Med 2010;17(1):11–7.

17. Soult MC, Weireter LJ, Britt RC, et al. Can routine trauma bay chest x-ray be bypassed with an extended focused assessment with sonography for trauma examination? Am Surg 2015;81(4):336–40.

18. Kong VY, Oosthuizen GV, Clarke DL. The selective conservative management of small traumatic pneumothoraces following stab injuries is safe: experience from a high-volume trauma service in South Africa. Eur J Trauma Emerg Surg 2015;41(1):75–9.

19. Zhang M, Teo LT, Goh MH, et al. Occult pneumothorax in blunt trauma: is there a need for tube thoracostomy? Eur J Trauma Emerg Surg 2016;2016:1863–9933.

20. Molnar TF. History of thoracic surgery ESTS textbook of thoracic surgery. In: Kuzdzal J, editor. Medycyna Praktyczna? Cracow (Poland); 2014. p. 3–33.

21. Abboud PA, Kendall J. Emergency department ultrasound for hemothorax after blunt traumatic injury. J Emerg Med 2003;25:181–4.

22. Molnar TF. Surgical management of chest wall trauma. Thorac Surg Clin 2010;20(4):475–85.

23. Griffiths JR, Roberts N. Do junior doctors know where to insert chest drains safely? Postgrad Med J 2005;81:456–8.

24. Laws D, Neville E, Duff J. British Thoracic Society guidelines for the insertion of a chest drain. Thorax 2003;58(Suppl II):ii53–9.

25. Tomlinson MA, Treasure T. Insertion of a chest drain: how to do it. Br J Hosp Med 1997;58:248–52.

26. Matsumoto S, Sekine K, Funabiki T, et al. Chest tube insertion direction: is it always necessary to insert a chest tube posteriorly in primary trauma care? Am J Emerg Med 2015;33(1):88–91.

27. Beckett A, Savage E, Pannell D, et al. Needle decompression for tension pneumothorax in Tactical Combat Casualty Care: do catheters placed in the midaxillary line kink more often than those in the midclavicular line? J Trauma 2011;71(5 Suppl 1):S408–12.

28. Inaba K, Lustenberger T, Recinos G, et al. Does size matter? A prospective analysis of 28-32 versus 36-40 French chest tube size in trauma. J Trauma Acute Care Surg 2012;72(2):422–7.

29. Kulvatunyou N, Joseph B, Friese RS, et al. 14 French pigtail catheters placed by surgeons to drain blood on trauma patients: is 14-Fr too small? J Trauma Acute Care Surg 2012;73(6):1423–7.

30. Kulvatunyou N, Erickson L, Vijayasekaran A, et al. Randomized clinical trial of pigtail catheter versus chest tube in injured patients with uncomplicated traumatic pneumothorax. Br J Surg 2014;101(2):17–22.

31. Kong VY, Clarke DL. The spectrum of visceral injuries secondary to misplaced intercostal chest drains: experience from a high volume trauma service in South Africa. Injury 2014;45(9):1435–9.

32. Kong VY, Oosthuizen GV, Sartorius B, et al. An audit of the complications of intercostal chest drain insertion in a high volume trauma service in South Africa. Ann R Coll Surg Engl 2014;96(8):609–13.

33. Harris A, O'Driscoll BR, Turkington PM. Survey of major complications of intercostal chest drain insertion in the UK. Postgrad Med J 2010;86(1012):68–72.

34. Bosman A, de Jong MB, Debeij J, et al. Systematic review and meta-analysis of antibiotic prophylaxis to prevent infections from chest drains in blunt and penetrating thoracic injuries. Br J Surg 2012;99(4):506–13.

35. Holzheimer R. Re: should we use routinely prophylactic antibiotics in patients with chest trauma?. Invited commentary. World J Surg 2006;30:2080–1.

36. Luketich JD, Kiss MD, Hershey J. Chest tube insertion: a prospective evaluation of pain management. Clin J Pain 1998;14:152–4.

37. Tang AT, Velissaris TJ, Weeded DF. An evidence-based approach to drainage of the pleural cavity: evaluation of best practice. J Eval Clin Pract 2002;8(3):333–40.

38. Howes RJ, Calder A, Hollingsworth A, et al. The end for the 'Roman Sandal': an observational study of methods of securing chest drains in a deployed military setting. J R Nav Med Serv 2015;101(1):42–6.

39. Inzirillo F, Giorgetta C, Ravalli E, et al. "Roman Sandal" modified method for securing the chest drain to the skin. Gen Thorac Cardiovasc Surg 2013;61(3):171–3.

40. Johnson CH, Lang SA, Bilal H, et al. In patients with extensive subcutaneous emphysema, which technique achieves maximal clinical resolution: infraclavicular incisions, subcutaneous drain insertion or suction on in situ chest drain? Interact Cardiovasc Thorac Surg 2014;18(6):825–9.

41. Peters J, Ketelaars R, van Wageningen B, et al. Prehospital thoracostomy in patients with traumatic circulatory arrest: results from a physician-staffed Helicopter Emergency Medical Service. Eur J Emerg Med 2015;2015:0969–9546.

42. Molnar TF, Rendeki SZ. Management of flail chest. In: Ferguson MK, editor. Difficult decisions in thoracic surgery. New York: Springer; 2014. p. 755–67.

43. Broder JS, Fox JW, Milne J, et al. Heimlich valve orientation error leading to radiographic tension pneumothorax: analysis of an error and a call for education, device redesign and regulatory action. Emerg Med J 2016;33(4):260–7.

44. Rigal S, Pous F. Triage of mass casualties in war conditions: realities and lessons learned. Int Orthop 2013;37(8):1433–8.

45. Wang HZ, Wu HY. Problems in the management of mass casualties in the Tian jin explosion. Crit Care 2016;20:47.

46. Hon HH, Elmously A, Stehly CD, et al. Inappropriate preinjury warfarin use in trauma patients: a call for a safety initiative. J Postgrad Med 2016;62(2):73–9.

Chest Tube Management after Surgery for Pneumothorax

Cecilia Pompili, MD[a], Michele Salati, MD[b],
Alessandro Brunelli, MD, FEBTS[a],*

KEYWORDS

- Pneumothorax • Bullectomy • Chest drainage • Suction • Pleurodesis

KEY POINTS

- Current evidence on the management of chest tubes after surgery for primary spontaneous pneumothorax is scarce.
- Current clinical practice is mostly based on personal experience and background or extrapolated from the literature on lung cancer surgery.
- The presence of a residual pleural space should be minimized to reduce the risk of recurrence.

MANAGEMENT OF CHEST TUBES AFTER LUNG RESECTION

Suction Versus No Suction

There are relative pros and cons in using suction versus no suction. Theoretically, suction promotes pleura-pleural apposition favoring the sealing of air leak and certainly favoring the drainage of large air leaks. However, suction has also been shown to increase the flow through the chest tube proportional to the level of suction applied[1] and it is assumed that this increased airflow increases the duration of drainage. Further, the use of suction has historically been associated with reduced patient mobilization, particularly if wall suction is used. On the other hand, the so-called no suction or alternate suction approaches have been shown to be effective in some circumstances to reduce the duration of air leak,[2–4] presumably by decreasing the air flow, while favoring mobilization (because the patient is not attached to the wall suction). Nonetheless, the absence of suction makes this approach ineffective in case of medium to large air leaks (particularly in the presence of a large pneumothorax)[2] and seems to be associated with an increased risk of other complications (particularly pneumonia and arrhythmia).[5]

Table 1 summary of the findings of the randomized trials published on suction versus no suction in lung resection subjects. These trials yielded mixed results. Some investigators found a benefit by using water seal,[2,3,7] others did not find any difference between the 2 modalities.[5,6]

The lack of objective data for more sensitive measurement of air leak severity has prevented the standardization of studies, and even test and control groups within studies, resulting in a lack of accurate quantification and reproducibility.

Regulated Suction

Some new electronic chest drainage systems are now able to measure the pleural pressure. There is scant evidence on the role of pleural pressure

---

Disclosure: Dr A. Brunelli and Dr C. Pompili have received in the past research grants and speaker honoraria from Medela Healthcare, Switzerland.

[a] Department of Thoracic Surgery, St. James's University Hospital, Beckett Street, Leeds LS9 7TF, UK; [b] Division of Thoracic Surgery, Ospedali Riuniti, Ancona, Italy
* Corresponding author.
E-mail address: brunellialex@gmail.com

Table 1
Summary of randomized trials comparing suction versus no suction after lung resection surgery

Author	Algorithm	Number of Subjects	Favor No Suction	Benefit
Cerfolio et al,[2] 2001	No suction on POD2	33	Yes	Larger air leak seal by POD3
Marshall et al,[3] 2002	No suction on ward arrival	68	Yes	Shorter air leak duration
Brunelli et al,[5] 2004	No suction on POD1	145	No	No difference in air leak duration, increased trend of complications
Brunelli et al,[4] 2005	Alternate suction	94	Yes to alternate suction	Shorter tube duration, LOS, less PAL vs full-time no suction
Alphonso et al,[6] 2005	Immediate no suction	234	No	No difference
Gocyk et al,[7] 2016	No suction on POD1	254	Yes	Shorter chest tube duration and reduced incidence of PAL in no suction subjects

Abbreviations: LOS, length of stay; PAL, prolonged air leak, POD, postoperative day.

on the healing of the lung parenchyma after surgery and duration of air leak.

A recent article has shown that the difference between minimum pressure and maximum pressure calculated from measurements taken during the sixth postoperative hour following lobectomy was associated with the duration of air leak and the risk of a prolonged air leak.[8] More than half of subjects with an airflow greater than 50 mL/min and a differential pressure greater than 10 cm H_2O developed an air leak longer than 3 days. Therefore, there seems to be the potential to influence the duration of air leak by altering the intrapleural pressure.

New digital drainage systems have the capability to deliver a regulated suction, which is a suction variable according to the feedback received from the pressure measurements to maintain the preset level of negative pressure. These machines work to maintain a stable intrapleural pressure regardless the volume of air leak, minimizing the oscillations around the preset value.

Modern chest drain devices, which are able to apply regulated suction to maintain the preset intrapleural pressure, represent the ideal instruments to reliably assess the effect of different level of negative pressures on the duration of air leak.[9] These may overcome the main limitation of previous trials using traditional devices and comparing suction versus no suction: the impossibility to control whether the preset level of suction was indeed maintained inside the chest.

In this regard, a recent randomized study assessed the effect of different levels of pleural pressure on the duration of air leak under controlled conditions by using a regulated chest drainage system.[10] One-hundred subjects who submitted to pulmonary lobectomy were randomized to receive 2 different types of chest drainage management. Group 1 received the regulated individualized suction mode, with different pressure levels depending on the type of lobectomy, and ranging from −11 cm H_2O to −20 cm H_2O based on a previous investigation.[11] Group 2 received regulated seal mode (−2 cm H_2O). At this low level of suction the system used worked only to compensate the occurrence of values more positive than −2 cm H_2O in case of air leak. Otherwise, it worked passively as a regulated, no-suction device. The average air leak duration and the number of subjects with prolonged air leak were similar between the groups, showing that regulated seal is as effective and safe as regulated suction in managing chest tubes following lobectomy.

More investigations are warranted to further clarify the role of intrapleural pressure on the recovery of lung parenchyma after surgery.

MANAGEMENT OF CHEST TUBES AFTER SURGERY FOR PNEUMOTHORAX
Suction Versus No Suction

There is scant evidence regarding the management of chest tubes after surgery for primary spontaneous pneumothorax (PSP). Although there seems to be consensus on the preferred surgical approach, video-assisted thoracic surgery (VATS), to perform bullectomy and pleurodesis, there are few studies investigating the effect of different drainage modalities on the occurrence of pneumothorax recurrence, which is the main outcome in these patients. Recent guidelines do not recommend the systematic use of suction in all patients treated for PSP but only in those who show failed lung re-expansion after drainage.[12,13]

It has been shown that the presence of a residual pleural space after surgery may be a factor associated with increased risk of recurrence. In a series of more than 400 subjects operated on for PSP or secondary spontaneous pneumothorax, Gaunt and colleagues[14] found an incidence of residual apical space after chest tube removal of 30%. Residual apical space was associated with 1 day longer duration of chest tube and 1 day longer hospital stay compared with those without residual apical space. More importantly, a residual apical space was the only factor associated with recurrence of pneumothorax after logistic regression analysis. Subjects with a residual apical space at discharge had an incidence of recurrence of 11.6% versus 4.4% of those without it ($P = .005$).

One possible hypothesis to explain the association between residual pleural space and recurrence of pneumothorax may be the failed pleurodesis due to lack of pleura-pleura apposition. The concept of applying suction to promote parietal to visceral pleura apposition and favoring the sealing of air leak by promoting pleurodesis is the same discussed in several studies comparing suction versus no suction after lobectomy.

Indeed, Varela and colleagues[15] have shown that applying suction to chest drainage after uncomplicated upper lobectomy can reduce the differential pleural pressure (difference between inspiratory and expiratory pressure values). This is likely explained by a reduction in volume of the residual apical pleural space, allowing for a decreased inspiratory pressure to achieve lung expansion. From this point of view, it seems logical to apply some level of negative pressure to the chest tube after bullectomy and pleurodesis operation for PSP.

A recent meta-analysis has shown no clear difference between suction and no suction in terms of air leak duration, chest tube duration, and hospital stay with very low level of evidence quality. The only endpoint with a moderate level of quality evidence was the reduction in the incidence of residual pneumothorax when suction is applied after lung resection.[16]

To the best of the authors' knowledge, there is only 1 study that compared suction versus no suction after bullectomy and pleurectomy for PSP. Ayed[17] randomized 100 subjects to either suction (−20 cm H$_2$O) or no suction after VATS bullectomy

and pleurodesis. They found that subjects managed with chest tube connected to suction had a 1 day longer chest tube duration and hospital stay, and higher incidence of prolonged air leak compared with those with chest tube managed without suction. In particular, those with suction had a prolonged air leak incidence of 14% versus 2% in those without suction ($P = .03$). The investigators reported only 2 recurrences of pneumothorax, too small a number to perform a reliable comparison between suction and no suction.

Regulated Suction and Recurrence

There is only 1 study evaluating the effect of the application of a regulating suction device in the management of chest tubes after bullectomy and pleurodesis for PSP.[18] This was a retrospective analysis that included 174 consecutive subjects operated on for PSP by uniportal VATS, and submitted to bullectomy and mechanical pleurodesis in 2 centers. Subjects' chest tubes were managed either by applying external wall suction for 48 hours or by using an electronic chest drainage system to deliver a regulated suction (variable suction to maintain a predetermined level of intrapleural pressure). To minimize selection bias, the investigators used propensity score case-matching analysis and compared 2 matched groups of 68 subjects. They found that the incidence of 1-year recurrence rate was more than 3-fold higher in the group managed with traditional suction compared with the group managed with regulated suction (14% vs 4.4%, $P = .04$). Moreover, the incidence of air leak duration, chest tube duration, and hospital stay was similar between the 2 groups.

Although a causal relationship cannot be proven with a retrospective analysis, it is possible that the application of a regulated suction can stabilize the intrapleural pressure, favoring pleura-pleura apposition and enhancing pleurodesis. In turn, this can lead to a reduction of pneumothorax recurrences.

Although this hypothesis is intriguing, further studies with clinical-pathologic models are warranted to better define the role of intrapleural pressure with the effect of pleurodesis.

Final Considerations

It seems clear that the current evidence on the management of chest tubes after surgery for PSP is scarce. Current clinical practice is mostly based on personal experience and background or extrapolated from the literature on lung cancer surgery.

The authors' personal preference in the management of chest tubes after minimally invasive surgery for PSP follows.

One 24 to 28 French single tube is used. Regulated suction is applied at a level of -20 cm H_2O for 48 hours to promote lung expansion and pleural juxtaposition favoring pleurodesis. If no air leak is present after 48 hours, the tube is removed following a chest radiograph to rule out the presence of a residual pleural space. Conversely, if an air leak is still present after 48 hours, the regulated suction is reduced from -20 cm H_2O to -8 cm H_2O to reduce the volume of air leak. In subjects with a persistent air leak (reported as 8% of the total in the literature), a trial with a portable device (Heimlich valve) can also be attempted after few days of drainage with suction at -8 cm H_2O, in preparation for discharge. However, one should always keep in mind that the presence of a residual pleural space should be minimized to reduce the risk of recurrence.

REFERENCES

1. Manzanet G, Vela A, Corell R, et al. A hydrodynamic study of pleural drainage systems: some practical consequences. Chest 2005;127(6):2211–21.

2. Cerfolio RJ, Bass C, Katholi CR. Prospective randomized trial compares suction versus water seal for air leaks. Ann Thorac Surg 2001;71(5):1613–7.

3. Marshall MB, Deeb ME, Bleier JI, et al. Suction vs water seal after pulmonary resection: a randomized prospective study. Chest 2002;121(3):831–5.

4. Brunelli A, Sabbatini A, Xiume' F, et al. Alternate suction reduces prolonged air leak after pulmonary lobectomy: a randomized comparison versus water seal. Ann Thorac Surg 2005;80(3):1052–5.

5. Brunelli A, Monteverde M, Borri A, et al. Comparison of water seal and suction after pulmonary lobectomy: a prospective, randomized trial. Ann Thorac Surg 2004;77(6):1932–7.

6. Alphonso N, Tan C, Utley M, et al. A prospective randomized controlled trial of suction versus non-suction to the under-water seal drains following lung resection. Eur J Cardiothorac Surg 2005; 27(3):391–4.

7. Gocyk W, Kuzdzal J, Wlodarczyk J, et al. Comparison of suction vs. non suction drainage after lung resections- a prospective randomized trial. Ann Thorac Surg 2016;102(4):1119–24.

8. Brunelli A, Cassivi SD, Salati M, et al. Digital measurements of air leak flow and intrapleural pressures in the immediate postoperative period predict risk of prolonged air leak after pulmonary lobectomy. Eur J Cardiothorac Surg 2011;39(4):584–8.

9. Brunelli A, Beretta E, Cassivi SD, et al. Consensus definitions to promote an evidence-based approach to management of the pleural space. A collaborative proposal by ESTS, AATS, STS, and GTSC. Eur J Cardiothorac Surg 2011;40(2):291–7.

10. Brunelli A, Salati M, Pompili C, et al. Regulated tailored suction vs regulated seal: a prospective randomized trial on air leak duration. Eur J Cardiothorac Surg 2013;43(5):899–904.

11. Refai M, Brunelli A, Varela G, et al. The values of intrapleural pressure before the removal of chest tube in non-complicated pulmonary lobectomies. Eur J Cardiothorac Surg 2012;41(4):831–3.

12. MacDuff A, Arnold A, Harvey J, BTS Pleural Disease Guideline Group. Management of spontaneous pneumothorax: British Thoracic Society Pleural Disease Guideline 2010. Thorax 2010;65(Suppl 2): ii18–31.

13. Baumann MH, Strange C, Heffner JE, et al. Management of spontaneous pneumothorax. ACCP Delphi Consensus Statement. Chest 2001;119:590–602.

14. Gaunt A, Martin-Ucar AE, Beggs L, et al. Residual apical space following surgery for pneumothorax increases the risk of recurrence. Eur J Cardiothorac Surg 2008;34(1):169–73.

15. Varela G, Brunelli A, Jiménez MF, et al. Chest drainage suction decreases differential pleural pressure after upper lobectomy and has no effect after lower lobectomy. Eur J Cardiothorac Surg 2010; 37(3):531–4.

16. Coughlin SM, Emmerton-Coughlin HM, Malthaner R. Management of chest tubes after pulmonary resection: a systematic review and meta-analysis. Can J Surg 2012;55(4):264–70.

17. Ayed AK. Suction versus water seal after thoracoscopy for primary spontaneous pneumothorax: prospective randomized study. Ann Thorac Surg 2003; 75:1593–6.

18. Pompili C, Xiumè F, Hristova R, et al. Regulated drainage reduces the incidence of recurrence after uniportal video-assisted thoracoscopic bullectomy for primary spontaneous pneumothorax: a propensity case-matched comparison of regulated and unregulated drainage. Eur J Cardiothorac Surg 2016; 49(4):1127–31.

Modern Techniques to Insert Chest Drains

Philip J. McElnay, MBChB, MRCS[a], Eric Lim, MBChB, MD, MSc, FRCS(C-Th)[a,b],*

KEYWORDS

- Chest tubes • Best practices • Procedure • Thoracic surgical • Training

KEY POINTS

- Chest drains are indicated in hemothorax, symptomatic pleural effusion, large or progressive pneumothorax, and postoperatively in thoracic surgery.
- They can be inserted using either "wide-bore" or Seldinger techniques. More recently, indwelling pleural catheters have been adopted for use in malignant pleural effusions.
- A chest drain can be associated with complications, such as hemothorax, organ perforation, empyema, and postremoval pneumothorax.
- After-care, including analgesia, monitoring, and chest radiographs, is vital to ensure their safe use.

INTRODUCTION

Nature of the Problem

Chest drains are inserted intraoperatively in thoracic surgery; however, they can be life saving in their own right in an acute situation. Independent indications include large or progressive pneumothorax, hemothorax, symptomatic pleural effusion, empyema, and chylothorax.[1]

However, they are invasive and can have potentially serious complications. Innovation now allows for insertion of drains, albeit of different calibers, via either Seldinger or surgical techniques.

Surgical Technique

There have been a myriad of advances over the past number of decades regarding the technique of chest drain insertion. Some of these include the following:

Surgical drain versus Seldinger drain

There has been a move in the last decade toward increasing use of Seldinger drains instead of "wide-bore" (also known as "surgical" or "argyle-type") drains.[2] Physicians frequently insert these in patients who have been admitted with an acute, symptomatic pleural effusion. It is worth noting that between 2003 and 2010 the Medicines and Healthcare Regulatory Authority reported 9 adverse incidents related to chest drain insertion (likely to be an underestimation of actual incidents), and all but one of them were related to Seldinger chest drains.[3] However, alternative reviews have suggested a much lower rate of complications associated with Seldinger drains compared with wide-bore drains (0.2% and 1.4%, respectively).[4] Specific risks associated with Seldinger drains include organ perforation by the dilators and drain blockage due to a narrower lumen.[5] There are many proposed benefits of Seldinger drains, such as increased patient comfort and ease or speed of insertion.[5] In fact, the British Thoracic Society now recommends use of Seldinger drains in spontaneous pneumothorax and malignant pleural effusion.[6,7]

The use of point-of-care ultrasound during drain insertion

Following initial investigation with chest radiology, chest drains have traditionally been inserted using

a Department of Cardiothoracic Surgery, James Cook University Hospital, Marton Road, Middlesbrough, TS4 3BW, UK; b Imperial College and the Academic Division of Thoracic Surgery, Royal Brompton Hospital, Sydney Street, London SW3 6NP, UK
* Corresponding author. Imperial College and the Academic Division of Thoracic Surgery, Royal Brompton Hospital, Sydney Street, London SW3 6NP, UK.
E-mail address: Eric.lim@imperial.ac.uk

Thorac Surg Clin 27 (2017) 29–34
http://dx.doi.org/10.1016/j.thorsurg.2016.08.005
1547-4127/17/© 2016 Elsevier Inc. All rights reserved.

clinical examination and anatomic landmarks alone. With the advent of Seldinger drains, the hope was that incorrect placement and organ injury may be reduced. However, following persistence in complication rates and the widespread availability of point-of-care ultrasound equipment, guidelines have moved toward recommending the use of insertion of drains under ultrasound guidance.[4]

Indwelling pleural catheters

Indwelling pleural catheters are now used routinely in the management of malignant pleural effusion in the United States and increasingly used elsewhere.[8] They involve "tunneling" a drain underneath the skin and into the pleural space. The tunneled nature of the tube and its associated cuff allows the drain to remain in situ for a longer period of time when compared with a wide-bore drain. The suggested benefits of indwelling pleural catheters (IPC) include management of the patient's condition at home and shorter hospital length of stay.[9] They are also progressively being used for other indications, such as hepatic hydrothorax and inflammatory pleuritis.[8]

Preoperative Planning

Many hospitals now use preformed packs of equipment for both Seldinger and surgical techniques. The clinician should, of course, ensure that these still contain all the required equipment before commencing.

To ensure safety, a chest radiograph should also be available before the procedure, and the diagnosis and laterality should be confirmed before starting the procedure.

Patients should be informed of the name of the procedure, what it involves, the potential benefits, serious and common potential complications, and alternative options. After providing the patient with sufficient information, informed consent should be sought and a written consent form completed.

There is often merit in providing the patient with some analgesia before the procedure, for example, oral morphine. This analgesia helps to ensure the patient is comfortable throughout the procedure.

Preparation and Patient Positioning

Insertion of a drain can be performed either intraoperatively or under local anesthesia if the condition does not require an operation. For the former, the patient is prepared according to the protocol of the respective operation. Here, preparation for the latter is discussed. Patients should

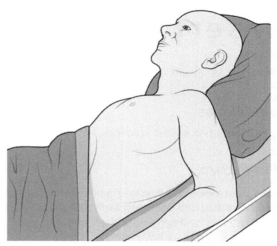

Fig. 1. The patient is positioned at a 45° angle on the bed. (*From* Lim E, Sadri A. Thorax. In: Novell R, editor. Kirk's general surgical operations. 6th edition. Philadelphia: Elsevier Inc.; 2013. p. 434–46; with permission.)

be in the supine position, with their torso raised to 45° on the bed (**Fig. 1**). They should be asked to place one hand (on the same side as the chest drain insertion) comfortably on the bed.

The ideal location for the insertion of the drain, to avoid vital structures, is within the "quadrangle of safety"—the borders of which are mid-axillary line (posterior limit), pectoral groove (anterior limit), and between the third and fifth intercostal space.[10] It can be helpful to mark a suitable position on the patient's chest before sterile preparation. Indeed, modern guidelines strongly recommend inserting chest drains under ultrasound guidance and go as far as to suggest that those inserting chest drains should receive formal training in ultrasonography for that purpose.[4]

The patient should be prepared with appropriate cleaning solutions, such as an iodine or chlorhexidine-based solution, and draped with sterile drapes, leaving only a small area around the point to be used for drain insertion exposed.

There are 2 main methods of drain insertion: a "wide-bore" (or "surgical") technique and a Seldinger technique. Both techniques are discussed later. All further steps as demonstrated later should be performed using a sterile technique.

Procedural Approach—Wide Bore

Step 1

After adequate preparation and positioning, the patient should have the chest anesthetized using a 3-level field block. A 3-level field block is done by inserting the needle into the intercostal space immediately above the chosen space, "walking the needle down the rib," angling the needle slightly superiorly and delivering approximately 2 mL of local anesthetic. The same technique should also be done for the chosen space and the space below the chosen space. A wheal of local anesthetic should also be created in the skin over the space where the chest drain is to be inserted.

Step 2
After being confident that local anesthetic has had adequate time to take effect, the clinician should make an incision with a sharp knife. It is common practice to use an "11-blade" knife. A common mistake is to make the skin incision too small. The skin incision should be large enough for the clinician to insert their finger into the chest. It is common for bleeding to occur at this stage, and if a swab is held on the wound after making the incision, it can maintain the patient's dignity, while minimizing infection risk. Place the knife back onto the sterile tray in a safe and visible position.

Step 3
Using a set of Roberts forceps, spread the subcutaneous tissues from the skin down to the rib. Spreading the subcutaneous tissues should be done in a safe manner by inserting the forceps in the closed position, gently opening them inside the patient, and closing them again before advancing. While gently advancing, open the forceps again. Caution must be taken as the forceps approach the rib not to advance rapidly into the patient's pleural cavity in an uncontrolled manner. Gently open the forceps above the rib to spread the tissue and gently advance while holding the forceps with both hands to ensure they are adequately controlled. As the forceps breach the pleura, there should be either a "whoosh of air" or the escape of fluid. At this point, remove the forceps and immediately place a finger in the wound.

Step 4
A finger sweep should be carried out, whereby the clinician places their index finger into the wound and gently sweeps around the wall of the thoracic cavity to confirm they are in the correct space (they should feel the smooth parietal pleura lining the wall of the thoracic cavity) and that no lung is adherent to the chest wall. The ability of the clinician to enter a finger confidently into the pleural cavity is perhaps the most important step. If a finger cannot easily enter into the pleural cavity, the tract is unlikely to be able to admit a chest drain.

Step 5
The drain should be advanced basally for pleural effusions or apically for pneumothoraces.

Step 6
The chest drain should be connected to an underwater seal drain immediately, and the drain bottle placed on the floor beside the patient.

Step 7
A simple interrupted stitch with a double-throw slipknot (**Fig. 2**) should be placed at the edge of the wound using a number 2 suture (either silk or a synthetic monofilament suture can be used) and then tied to the drain to ensure it is secured in place. A knot that makes an indentation in the tube is adequately tight. An adhesive dressing is placed over the wound site.

Seldinger Technique

In recent years, the Seldinger technique has been adopted to insert chest drains in those who have uncomplicated pneumothoraces and nonloculated effusions. For apical pneumothoraces, insertion in the second intercostal space in the midclavicular line should be considered. For effusions, insertion should be in the "quadrangle of safety" as described above. The technique is also different to the "wide-bore" method:

Step 1
In a similar way to the "wide-bore" technique, after adequate preparation and positioning, the patient should have the chest anesthetized with local anesthetic. The needle is inserted down to the pleural space, aspirating with progression to ensure the needle is in the correct place. The needle should be inserted superiorly over the rib to ensure avoidance of the neurovascular bundle, which lies inferiorly to each rib along its course. After ensuring the needle is not in a blood vessel, the local anesthetic is injected to anesthetize the pleura, and a further local anesthetic is injected as the needle is withdrawn. The anesthetic should be allowed time to take effect to ensure the skin and underlying tissues are anesthetized.

Step 2
After being confident that local anesthetic has been infiltrated to the correct space and level and having left adequate time for local anesthetic to take effect, the clinician should then insert a wide-bore needle connected to a 10-mL syringe in the same plane as the previously inserted needle, aspirating as it is advanced. The needle should be inserted above the rib to avoid the neurovascular bundle. When air or fluid is aspirated again, the clinician should stop advancing the needle.

Step 3
The needle should be carefully held in place while the syringe is removed from the needle. After

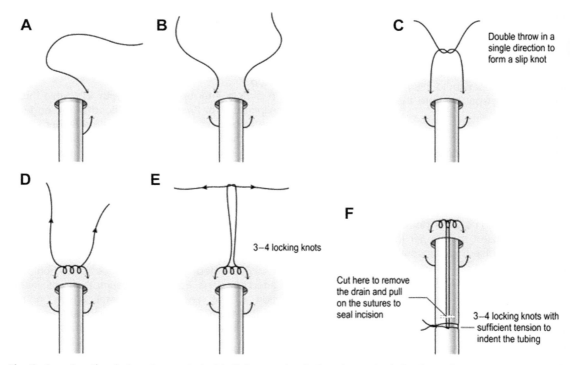

Fig. 2. Securing the drain using a stitch. (*A, B*) Secure the drain using a single horizontal mattress stitch. (*C, D*) A double throw secures the initial tie. (*E*) The knot is locked with 3-4 locking throws. (*F*) The stitch is secured to the drain using 3-4 knots sufficiently tight to indent the tubing. (*From* Lim E, Sadri A. Thorax. In: Novell R, editor. Kirk's general surgical operations. 6th edition. Philadelphia: Elsevier Inc.; 2013. p. 434–46; with permission.)

removing the syringe, a guidewire is inserted through the needle until approximately 20 cm of wire remains outside the patient. At this point, no further guidewire should be inserted inside the patient. The guidewire should be held securely in the same position at all times while the needle is removed from the patient over the wire. Under no circumstances should the wire be fully inserted into the chest; this would require emergency removal of the wire with an operation. To avoid this, the wire should be held firmly by the clinician at all times.

Step 4

The clinician should make an incision perpendicular to but very close to the wire with a scalpel. It is common practice to use an "11-blade" knife. The Seldinger technique is slightly different than the wide-bore technique in that it requires a short, sharp insertion motion of the scalpel rather than making a linear incision. A short, sharp insertion motion allows the creation of a skin incision that is just large enough for the insertion of the Seldinger drain over the wire.

Step 5

The clinician should then use sequentially larger "dilators" to increase the size of the track in the patient's subcutaneous tissues. Caution must be exercised to ensure the dilators are not inserted hastily or so far as to injure the patient's lung.

Step 6

The chest drain can then be inserted over the wire into the patient's pleural cavity. The distance to the pleural cavity will vary depending on the patient, but there should always be several centimeters of drain outside the patient's chest. When the drain is safely inside the pleural cavity, the wire can be removed. A finger should be placed over the end of the drain between removing the wire and picking up the next piece of equipment.

Step 7

A 3-way valve can be connected to the drain, which can then be connected to an unwater seal drain as per the wide-bore technique.

Step 8

A simple interrupted stitch can be placed at the edge of the wound using a number 2 suture (either silk or a synthetic monofilament suture can be used) and then tied to the drain to ensure it is secured in place. An adhesive dressing is placed over the wound site. Alternatively, Seldinger drains are sometimes secured using adhesive dressings alone, but this can be less secure and risks accidental drain removal.

Immediate Postprocedural Care

The postprocedural care following insertion of either wide-bore or Seldinger drains is comparable. Both groups should be provided with adequate analgesia and should receive a chest radiograph following the procedure. The chest radiograph allows assessment of lung inflation as well as assesses chest drain positioning.

REHABILITATION AND RECOVERY

The procedure of inserting a chest drain can be painful. After the procedure, the chest drain pain can continue, and it can be irritating to the visceral pleura and stimulate coughing. The patient should be reassured that this should settle after a short period of time. Analgesia should be given as required.

Ideally, 2 people should carry out drain removal: one to steadily remove the chest drain and the second to cover the skin incision with an adhesive dressing. Drains should be removed at either maximal inspiration or maximal expiration, with the patient holding their breath at either extreme, thus preventing air being entrained into the pleural space.

As the patient's breath is held, the drain should be removed in a single steady motion, with the second person immediately covering the drain site with the adhesive dressing.

It may be helpful to ask the patient to practice holding their breath at maximal inspiration or expiration 2 or 3 times before the removal of the drain.

CLINICAL RESULTS IN THE LITERATURE

Chest drains are inserted frequently in the hospital setting. However, population results are poorly reported in the literature, and studies are limited to small trials. Harris and colleagues[3] conducted one of the largest studies of complications following chest drain insertion. A survey was conducted among UK hospitals of complications associated with chest drains from 2003 to 2008. The authors received results from 101 of 148 acute hospital trusts. Over the study period, 20 Seldinger drains and 11 wide-bore drains were inserted on the wrong side, 3 wires were lost within the pleural space as part of the Seldinger technique, and 33 lung injuries were caused as a result of Seldinger drains and 9 as a result of wide-bore drains. There were 10 mortalities in the Seldinger group and 5 in the wide-bore group. While the study does not provide a denominator for the number of drains inserted, it does provide an overview of the potential complications associated with both types of drains. However, given the 5-year timeframe and potentially large population included in the survey, chest drains remain an acceptable and safe procedure.

The TIME2 trial is one of the most significant (n = 106) to have compared IPC with chest drain insertion and talc pleurodesis for patients with malignant pleural effusions.[11] It demonstrated no difference in dyspnea between the groups in the first 42 days, but a significant improvement in dyspnea in the IPC group at 6 months. Median IPC patient length of stay was shorter (0 days) compared with the talc group (4 days). Twelve patients in the talc group and 3 in the IPC group required further pleural procedures ($P = .03$). Twenty-one patients suffered an adverse event in the IPC group compared with 7 in the talc group ($P = .002$).

POTENTIAL COMPLICATIONS/MANAGEMENT

Patients who have had chest drains inserted are at risk of several complications. These complications can be divided into early and late complications:

Early

I. *Hemothorax.* This can be as a result of laceration to an intercostal blood vessel. It is a potentially serious complication and may require an emergency thoracotomy. There have also been reports of iatrogenic injury to the left ventricle following chest drain insertion, which requires emergency intervention via thoracotomy or sternotomy.[12]

II. *Lung laceration.* This can be as a result of over-insertion of a dilator in the Seldinger technique or by use of a trochar in wide-bore drain insertion.

III. Placement in the incorrect anatomic position
   a. *Abdominal.* This can happen with either wide-bore or Seldinger drains. Of particular concern is the perforation to abdominal viscera that can result from this error.
   b. *Subcutaneously.* The placement of a drain subcutaneously is a particular complication of Seldinger drains whereby the wire can be fed progressively and erroneously into the subcutaneous tissues, followed by the chest drain.

IV. *Pain.* This is a recognized complication following both types of drain. The procedure can be particularly painful if the drain is inserted too far.

V. *Inadvertent drain removal.* This can happen if the drain is not secured in place adequately.

Late

I. *Lumen blockage.* This can occur with either drain but is a particular risk in narrow lumen drains, such as those used in the Seldinger technique.
II. *Retained Hemothorax.* If a hemothorax is not adequately drained initially, it can clot and become impossible to drain via a chest drain. In addition, it can act as a locus of infection and result in empyema.
III. *Pneumothorax.* This can occur when poor technique is used to remove the drain, and air is entrained into the pleural space via the skin incision.

SUMMARY

Chest drains remain a vital and potentially life-saving part of thoracic and respiratory care. There have been several advances in their use, including the development of Seldinger techniques and IPC. They can be associated with significant risks such as hemothorax, organ perforation, and empyema; however, these can be minimized by following a meticulous technique.

REFERENCES

1. Dev S, Nascimiento B, Simone C, et al. Chest tube insertion. N Engl J Med 2007;357:e15.
2. Lee YC, Baumann MH, Maskell NA, et al. Pleurodesis practice for malignant pleural effusions in five English-speaking countries: survey of pulmonologists. Chest 2003;124:2229–38.
3. Harris A, O'Driscoll BR, Turkington PM. Survey of major complications of intercostal chest drain insertion in the UK. Postgrad Med J 2010;86:68–72.
4. Havelock T, Teoh R, Laws D, et al, on behalf of the BTS Pleural Disease Guideline Group. Pleural procedures and thoracic ultrasound: British Thoracic Society Pleural Disease Guideline 2010. Thorax 2010;65(Suppl 2):ii61–76.
5. Maskell NA, Medford A, Gleeson FV. Seldinger chest drain insertion: simpler but not necessarily safer. Thorax 2010;65:5–6.
6. Henry M, Arnold T, Harvey J. BTS guidelines for the management of spontaneous pneumothorax. Thorax 2003;58(Suppl 2):ii39–52.
7. Antunes G, Neville E, Duffy J, et al. BTS guidelines for the management of malignant pleural effusions. Thorax 2003;58(Suppl 2):ii29–38.
8. Bhatnagar R, Reid ED, Corcoran JP, et al. Indwelling pleural catheters for non-malignant effusions: a multicentre review of practice. Thorax 2014;69(10):959–61.
9. Boshuizen RC, Thomas R, Lee YCG. Advantages of indwelling pleural catheters for management of malignant pleural effusions. Curr Respir Care Rep 2013;2:93–9.
10. British Thoracic Society Pleural Disease Guideline. 2010. Available at: https://www.brit-thoracic.org.uk/document-library/clinical-information/pleural-disease/pleural-disease-guidelines-2010/pleural-disease-guideline-quick-reference-guide/. Accessed February 15, 2016.
11. Davies HE, Mishra EK, Kahan BC. Effect of an indwelling pleural catheter vs chest tube and talc pleurodesis for relieving dyspnea in patients with malignant pleural effusion. JAMA 2012;307(22):2383–9.
12. Kim D, Lim SH, Seo PW. Iatrogenic perforation of the left ventricle during insertion of a chest drain. Korean J Thorac Cardiovasc Surg 2013;46(3):223–5.

Suction or Nonsuction
How to Manage a Chest Tube After Pulmonary Resection

Gaetano Rocco, MD, FRCSEd, FEBTS[a],*,
Alessandro Brunelli, MD, FEBTS[b], Raffaele Rocco, MD[c]

KEYWORDS

• Air leak • Chest drain • Chest tube • Lobectomy • Suction

KEY POINTS

• The dilemma as to whether to apply suction after subtotal pulmonary resection has not been solved.
• The problem lies in the poorly understood pathophysiology of the air leak phenomenon and the inadequate quality of the published randomized trials.
• Even digital systems do not seem to have made the difference.
• The authors propose an air leak predictor score as a contributing step toward appropriateness in using intraoperative sealants and chest tube management.

INTRODUCTION

Before wondering whether we should manage air leaks with suction or not, several issues must be taken for granted. As an example, a thorough evaluation of both the imaged and functional profile of the residual lung, the expertise of the surgeon (often related to his or her seniority in practice),[1] as well as the resort to a meticulous intraoperative surgical technique (inclusive of available sealants) to avoid air leaks represent milestones in effecting the quality of lung surgery.[2,3] If the aforementioned factors are excluded, an air leak developing after an uncomplicated lobectomy is usually a self-limiting phenomenon. This point means that a well-drained chest cavity after subtotal pulmonary resection will eventually lead to full re-expansion of the residual lung. Can this process be made more efficient and rapid to facilitate patient fast-tracking? Can we identify before surgery that 8% to 26% of patients who will end up after day 5 to

7 with a prolonged air leak (PAL)?[2] When faced with the dilemma of whether to apply suction in the immediate postoperative period, the thoracic surgeon still acts according to the need of preserving his or her peace of mind. Building science around this topic has involved the work of several contributors who have designed clinical research projects but found no real answer to the dilemma.[4,5] Recent meta-analysis and randomized trials provide suggestions but no real clue as to whether we will be able to one day individualize chest drain management (hence, suction) with an aim to reduce length of stay in the hospital.[3,5–10] So, what is next?

THE CONCEPT OF SUCTION

Miserocchi and coworkers[11] have authoritatively explained the concept of suction applied to a chest drain. In brief, they distinguished the suction generated by the height of the collecting reservoir

Disclosure Statement: Dr G. Rocco discloses a financial interest with Baxter Healthcare; Dr A. Brunelli discloses a financial interest with Medela Healthcare.
a Division of Thoracic Surgical Oncology, Department of Thoracic Surgical and Medical Oncology, Istituto Nazionale Tumori, Pascale Foundation, IRCCS, Naples, Italy; b Department of Thoracic Surgery, St. James's University Hospital, Leeds, UK; c Section of Thoracic Surgery, University Campus Biomedico, Rome, Italy
* Corresponding author.
E-mail address: g.rocco@istitutotumori.na.it

Thorac Surg Clin 27 (2017) 35–40
http://dx.doi.org/10.1016/j.thorsurg.2016.08.006

relative to the location of the tip of the chest drain from the suction generated by an external device.[11] Accordingly, a water seal provides a suction pressure, the extent of which strictly depends on the described height difference.[11] Based on this definition, we should not be comparing suction with no suction but rather external suction-to-suction pressure obtained from a height gradient.[11] In other words, the relevant question is as follows: Should we apply additional suction to the collection chamber in the face of a self-limiting phenomenon as routine postoperative air leak?

THE EVIDENCE FOR APPLYING (EXTERNAL/ ADDITIONAL) SUCTION

Since the early 2000s, several randomized controlled trials (RCTs) have been designed to compare suction with water seal.[7] Interestingly enough, the results did not support suction, showing either no difference or a definitive benefit only from no suction/water seal.[4–7] The institutional policy was to apply suction for the first night after surgery in all trials but one in which the suction was not applied at all in the postoperative period.[4–7] Based on the described physiology of suction applied to chest drain, the results from these RCTs are consistent with the idea that no additional suction is needed for routine postoperative air leaks.[4–7] The issue of whether additional suction is needed for patients at risk of developing PALs is still debated.[12] In fact, increasing the intrapleural negative pressure by applying external/additional suction is seen as potentially detrimental because it may worsen the extent or the duration of an alveolo-pleural fistula.[12] In 2012, Coughlin and associates[12] authored an elegant meta-analysis of the available contributions in the literature comparing external/additional suction plus water seal with a water seal alone in an effort to avoid PALs. The design of this study acknowledged the existence, in the water-seal setting, of an intrathoracic suction pressure originating from the height difference between the tip of the chest drain and the level of the collection chamber and that an external suction device provides, if necessary, additional suction pressure.[12] Overall, 7 RCTs published between 2001 and 2008 were considered, including series ranging between 31 and 254 patients.[12] In spite of a low or very low quality of the studies included in the meta-analysis, the absence of a publication bias was demonstrated by funnel plot symmetry.[12] However, a major source of concern was the different definition of PALs that varied from 3 to more than 7 days.[12] The analysis demonstrated a trend toward reduction and duration of PALs with a water seal; subgroup analysis, used to avoid heterogeneity, demonstrated that the effect on the air leak incidence could be reliable for air leaks lasting more than 6 days.[12] In addition, if outlier studies were removed from the analysis along with the adoption of a fixed-effects model, other outcomes, such as duration of air leak and time to discharge, favored a water seal.[12] Conversely, additional suction was a major determinant in reducing postoperative pneumothorax, although this did not translate into a decreased duration of chest drain and hospitalization.[12] The investigators concluded that no inference could be drawn from the meta-analysis in terms of comparison of water seal versus suction and that higher-quality and larger-numbered RCTs need to be designed in the future to finally address this issue.[12] Overlapping conclusions were reached by Qiu and coworkers[13] in a meta-analysis published in 2013 whereby no difference as to primary and secondary outcomes was observed between external suction and water seal. Lang and colleagues[3] have more recently published an interesting review on the discordance between clinical practice and literature evidence on the use of suction for postoperative air leaks. This meta-analysis encompassed a larger number of patients and the evaluation of additional RCTs compared with previous studies.[3] Compared with previous findings, the striking feature of this article is the detection of a statistically significant difference favoring water seal over external suction in terms of air leak and chest drain duration as well as length of stay in the hospital.[3] As expected, no predominance of one treatment over the other was seen when the effect on the incidence of PALs was considered, whereas the value of suction in reducing postoperative pneumothorax was confirmed.[3] The same study also included a survey of the clinical use of suction in the postoperative period in the UK thoracic surgical units that demonstrated a significant variability in the clinical practice in the absence of a grade IA evidence to direct the treatment choice.[3]

THE ROLE OF DIGITAL DRAIN SYSTEMS

Reportedly, digital drain systems contribute to the mobilization of patients who are freed from the wall suction and provide continuous and objective air leak monitoring which, in turn, may facilitate early detection of cessation of the air leak, thereby prompting chest drain removal.[3,14,15] With these devices, fast-tracking becomes possible, albeit their costs need to be carefully weighed against the aforementioned benefits.[3] In 2014, Afoke and colleagues[16] published a review based on the best available evidence on the use of digital drain systems with special focus on the impact on drain removal. Interestingly, all series originated from single-institution studies and included patients with acceptable pulmonary function.[16] The investigators concluded that the heterogeneity of the different studies in terms of type and number of drain systems considered, duration of hospitalization, and inclusion of cost estimates prevented them from drawing meaningful conclusions in favor of the routine use of such devices.[16] In this setting, Varela and coworkers have supported the implementation of a well-defined air leak predictive model to eliminate a significant interobserver variability and possibly obviate digital drain systems.[17] Recently, a multicenter randomized trial compared the use of digital versus traditional drain systems in terms of timing of chest drain removal and patient satisfaction.[18] This study included 381 patients undergoing lobectomy and segmentectomy managed through an equal share of traditional and digital chest drain systems of the same manufacturer with the latter associated with a statistically significant reduction of air leak, chest drain, and hospital stay duration.[18] In addition, subjective data showed increased patient satisfaction expressed with a perceived improved ability mobilization, user friendliness of the device, and confidence in being dismissed home on the digital drain system.[18] Important limitations were acknowledged because this investigator-initiated study was unblinded to both patients and researchers and a cost analysis could not be performed.[18] In this setting, important issues with the statistical design and methodology as well as the calculation of the sample size of prospective randomized trials may potentially represent misleading factors in reaching reproducible conclusions.[19,20]

PREDICTING PROLONGED AIR LEAKS AND NEED FOR EXTERNAL SUCTION

One way to address the issue of when to apply the external suction depends on the ability to predict the onset of PALs. In the past, scoring systems and predictive models have been proposed with alternate fortune while interesting fields of research are currently being investigated.[21] As an example, in order to associate the extent of bubbling from traditional chest drains and need for external suction, Cerfolio and colleagues[22] devised a score that correlated a greater than 3 air leak score and a pneumothorax greater than 8 cm to the need for restoring suction.

In this setting, the presence of pleural hypercarbia has been suggested to correlate with the duration of air leaks.[23] In a recent study, Bharat and colleagues[23] concluded that the evidence of pleural hypercarbia (ie, P_{CO_2} >6%) warrants the application of suction and oxygen supplementation in order to shorten the duration of the air leaks, whereas, in the absence of pleural hypercarbia, patients can be kept on water seal.

Prediction of compromised expiratory flow has been obtained through the assessment of volatile organic compound fingerprints with an electronic nose.[24] Although the study is preliminary, the possibility to use such a device in the decision-making process for external suction is more than an intriguing perspective.[24]

SUCTION STRATEGY

During the years, the use of traditional chest drain systems has ben associated with the need for a user-friendly model of interpretation of the air leak phenomenon in order to facilitate prompt chest drain removal and, therefore, impact hospitalization and costs.[25] The objective data available from digital drain systems have enabled physicians and nurses to minimize interobserver variability and reduce delays in the decision-making process for chest drain removal.[26] However, somehow in contradiction with previous findings from the same group,[27] a recent study from Salamanca clearly demonstrates that a model based on the interpretation of clinical variables in association with an air leak score measured via a traditional chest drain system may also effectively reduce interobserver variability of chest drain management after standard pulmonary resections.[17] Nevertheless, the ability to design a reproducible suction strategy is affected by the low level of quality of the available evidence in the literature to the point that Coughlin and colleagues[12] concluded that definitive recommendations as to chest tube management could not be issued and that an adequately powered RCT was warranted. In this setting, a complication grading system related to the development of PALs should be devised. As an example, the group from Ottawa adopted the Clavien classification system that, for PALs, defines grade II as the complication grade, which requires a chest tube for more than 5 days after surgery.[28,29] Moreover, grade III contemplates the insertion of an additional chest tube (grade IIIA) or reoperation (grade IIIB), whereas grades IV and V result in intensive care with life support and mortality within 30 days, respectively.[2] Hence, the use of a flutter bag or a Heimlich valve by itself is considered a grade II complication.[2] Accordingly, suction strategies should be compared based on their impact on maintaining the extent of the PAL complication within grade II of the Clavien score system.[2] Looking at the predictive model for PAL developed from the French Epithor Database, the risk group corresponding to the 7% PAL cutoff recorded in the database entails a moderate to low possibility of developing PALs[30]; in this risk category, the grade II Clavien PALs could also be included.

THE AIR LEAK PREDICTOR SCORE AS A PREDICTIVE TOOL FOR PROLONGED AIR LEAKS

The authors propose a literature-based score, which has been structured by using the indeed few reports expressing the most common predictors for PAL weighed either through odd risk (OR) values or logistic regression coefficients, which were also converted in OR values for the purpose of this analysis (OR = e$^{\text{regression coefficient}}$). With the aim to develop an aggregate score, the authors averaged the ORs of the risk factors reported in the principal studies assessing the risk of PAL after lobectomy by using logistic regression analysis. The mean of the ORs for each predictor was calculated. The PAL predictor with the lowest mean OR value was assigned the score of 1, and proportionally increasing scores have been attributed to the other predictors (**Table 1**). This score system needs to be validated in a forthcoming research project to test user friendliness,

effectiveness in reducing inappropriate use of suction and Clavien class II PALs.

Accordingly, a strategy to predict PAL and individualize possible application of suction in the postoperative period should be determined according to the following steps:

1. Retrospectively evaluate the PAL phenomenon (PALs longer than 5 days) from the institutional database; the resulting rate should be in the range of internationally accepted figures (ie, 5% to 13%[30]). If the figures are higher, a thorough analysis of the case mix, the surgical technique, and the need of intraoperative measures to abate the excessive rates of PALs must be carefully contemplated.
2. In this setting, the authors propose the adoption of a new air leak predictor score (ALPS; see **Table 1**) based on the following:
   a. Analyzing the risk factors reported in the literature possibly present in each patient
   b. Attributing each patient to a risk group by determining an individual score
      ALPS will be retrospectively validated on multicentric series in order to find the score cutoff beyond which advising on the following:
      i. The intraoperative use of lung sealants (Randomized trials will then be structured to test the efficacy of ALPS.)
      ii. Chest tube management by applying suction (ie, −20 cmH$_2$O) in the immediate 12 hours after surgery
      iii. The use of unidirectional valves (ie, Heimlich/flutter bags) to discharge patients home if with PALs

SUMMARY

The empirical approach to air leaks and chest tube management in the postoperative period has been a distinctive feature of the mastery of the art possessed by the senior thoracic surgeons. Many of us can narrate anecdotes of old mentors removing chest drains while there was some bubbling on coughing in the glass reservoir and the lung was not fully re-expanded on chest radiograph. Others may remember the times when no chest drain was removed before a 24-hour trial of provocative clamping. Nowadays, the ever-increasing knowledge of the pathophysiology beyond postoperative air leakage and the use of digital drain systems have made chest tube management progressively more a science and less an art.[31–33] Nevertheless, the jury is still out as to whether routine suction should be applied in the immediate postoperative period, with no final

---

Table 1
The relationship between the acknowledged risk factors for prolonged air leaks and a tailored approach to suction after subtotal anatomic lung surgery

Variables	OR	ALPS
Age >65 y	2.8	1.5
FEV$_1$ <80%	2.05 (1.9)	1.0
Male sex	3.47 (2.8)	2.0
Pl adhesions	2.86	1.5
BMI <25.5	2.8 (BMI <18.5: 2.6)	1.5
Upper lobe	1.89	1.0
Right side	4.46	2.0

The score cutoff to suggest the intraoperative use of sealants and an optimal chest tube management will be the object of further studies.

Abbreviations: ALPS, air leak predictor score; BMI, body mass index; FEV$_1$, forced expiratory volume in the first second of expiration; Pl, pleural.

Data from Refs.[2,4,15,30,32,33]

evidence resulting from the literature. The old dilemma "suction or no suction" cannot be solved for now.[12]

REFERENCES

1. Okereke I, Murthy SC, Alster JM, et al. Characterization and importance of air leak after lobectomy. Ann Thorac Surg 2005;79:1167–73.
2. Liang S, Ivanovic J, Gilbert S, et al. Quantifying the incidence and impact of postoperative prolonged alveolar air leak after pulmonary resection. J Thorac Cardiovasc Surg 2013;145(4):948–54.
3. Lang P, Manickavasagar M, Burdett C, et al. Suction on chest drains following lung resection: evidence and practice are not aligned. Eur J Cardiothorac Surg 2016;49:611–6.
4. Brunelli A, Monteverde M, Borri A, et al. Comparison of water seal and suction after pulmonary lobectomy: a prospective, randomized trial. Ann Thorac Surg 2004;77:1932–7.
5. Cerfolio R, Bass C, Katholi C. Prospective randomized trial compares suction versus water seal for air leaks. Ann Thorac Surg 2001;71:1613–7.
6. Marshall MB, Deeb ME, Bleier JIS, et al. Suction vs water seal after pulmonary resection—a randomized prospective study. Chest 2002;121:831–5.
7. Alphonso N, Tan C, Utley M, et al. A prospective randomized controlled trial of suction versus non-suction to the under-water seal drains following lung resection. Eur J Cardiothorac Surg 2005;27:391–4.
8. Brunelli A, Salati M, Refai M, et al. Evaluation of a new chest tube removal protocol using digital air leak monitoring after lobectomy: a prospective randomised trial. Eur J Cardiothorac Surg 2010;37:56–60.
9. Deng B, Tan QY, Zhao YP, et al. Suction or non-suction to the underwater seal drains following pulmonary operation: meta-analysis of randomised controlled trials. Eur J Cardiothorac Surg 2010;38:210–5.
10. Leo F, Duranti L, Girelli L, et al. Does external pleural suction reduce prolonged air leak after lung resection? Results from the AirINTrial after 500 randomized cases. Ann Thorac Surg 2013;96:1234–9.
11. Miserocchi G, Beretta E, Rivolta I. Respiratory mechanics and fluid dynamics after lung resection surgery. Thorac Surg Clin 2010;20:345–57.
12. Coughlin SM, Emmerton-Coughlin HMA, Malthaner R. Management of chest tubes after pulmonary resection: a systematic review and meta-analysis. Can J Surg 2012;55:264–70.
13. Qiu T, Shen Y, Wang MZ, et al. External suction versus water seal after selective pulmonary resection for lung neoplasm: systematic review. PLoS One 2013;8(7):e68087.
14. McGuire AL, Petrich W, Maziak DE, et al. Digital versus analogue pleural drainage phase 1: prospective evaluation of interobserver reliability in the assessment of pulmonary air leaks. Interact Cardiovasc Thorac Surg 2015;21:403–7.
15. Brunelli A, Varela G, Refai M, et al. A scoring system to predict the risk of prolonged air leak after lobectomy. Ann Thorac Surg 2010;90:204–9.
16. Afoke J, Tan C, Hunt I, et al. Might digital drains speed up the time to thoracic drain removal? Interact Cardiovasc Thorac Surg 2014;19:135–8.
17. Rodríguez M, Jiménez MF, Hernández MT, et al. Usefulness of conventional pleural drainage systems to predict the occurrence of prolonged air leak after anatomical pulmonary resection. Eur J Cardiothorac Surg 2015;48:612–5.
18. Pompili C, Detterbeck F, Papagiannopoulos K, et al. Multicenter international randomized comparison of objective and subjective outcomes between electronic and traditional chest drainage systems. Ann Thorac Surg 2014;98:490–6.
19. Gilbert S, McGuire AL, Maghera S, et al. Randomized trial of digital versus analog pleural drainage in patients with or without a pulmonary air leak after lung resection. J Thorac Cardiovasc Surg 2015;150:1243–51.
20. Lim E. The devil is in the details: managing chest drains and interpreting negative randomized trial data. J Thorac Cardiovasc Surg 2015;150:1252–3.
21. Lee L, Hanley SC, Robineau C, et al. Estimating the risk of prolonged air leak after pulmonary resection using a simple scoring system. J Am Coll Surg 2011;212:1027–32.
22. Cerfolio RJ, Bass CS, Pask AH, et al. Predictors and treatment of persistent air leaks. Ann Thorac Surg 2002;73:1727–30.
23. Bharat A, Graf N, Mullen A, et al. Pleural hypercarbia after lung surgery is associated with persistent alveolopleural fistulae. Chest 2016;149:220–7.
24. Incalzi RA, Pennazza G, Scarlata S, et al. Reproducibility and respiratory function correlates of exhaled breath fingerprint in chronic obstructive pulmonary disease. PLoS One 2012;7:e45396.
25. Martin-Ucar AE, Passera E, Vaughan R, et al. Implementation of a user-friendly protocol for interpretation of air-leaks and management of intercostal chest drains after thoracic surgery. Interact Cardiovasc Thorac Surg 2003;2:251–5.
26. Brunelli A, Cassivi SD, Salati M, et al. Digital measurements of air leak flow and intrapleural pressures in the immediate postoperative period predict risk of prolonged air leak after pulmonary lobectomy. Eur J Cardiothorac Surg 2011;39:584–8.
27. Varela G, Jiménez MF, Novoa NM, et al. Postoperative chest tube management: measuring air leak using an electronic device decreases variability in the clinical practice. Eur J Cardiothorac Surg 2009;35:28–31.

28. Ivanovic J, Al-Hussaini A, Al-Shehab D, et al. Evaluating the reliability and reproducibility of the Ottawa thoracic morbidity and mortality classification system. Ann Thorac Surg 2011;91:387–93.

29. Seely AJ, Ivanovic J, Threader J, et al. Systematic classification of morbidity and mortality after thoracic surgery. Ann Thorac Surg 2010;90:936–42.

30. Rivera C, Bernard A, Falcoz PE, et al. Characterization and prediction of prolonged air leak after pulmonary resection: a nationwide study setting up the index of prolonged air leak. Ann Thorac Surg 2011;92:1062–8.

31. Merritt RE, Singhal S, Shrager JB. Evidence-based suggestions for management of air leaks. Thorac Surg Clin 2010;20:435–48.

32. Petrella F, Rizzo S, Radice D, et al. Predicting prolonged air leak after standard pulmonary lobectomy: computed tomography assessment and risk factors stratification. Surgeon 2011;9:72–7.

33. Elsayed H, McShane J, Shackcloth M. Air leaks following pulmonary resection for lung cancer: is it a patient or surgeon related problem? Ann R Coll Surg Engl 2012;94:422–7.

When to Remove a Chest Tube

Nuria M. Novoa, MD, PhD*, Marcelo F. Jiménez, MD, PhD, EBCTS,
Gonzalo Varela, MD, PhD, EBCTS

KEYWORDS

- Postoperative air leak • Water seal drainage • Digital pleural drainage • Electronic pleural drainage
- Large pleural drainage • Daily output of pleural fluid

KEY POINTS

- Chest tube removal at the end of expiration with a stable Valsalva maneuver decreases the occurrence of clinically significant pneumothorax after pulling up drainages.
- Digital drainage systems allow differentiation of persisting air leak from pleural space effects when high differential pleural pressure and expiratory bubbling occurs.
- Digital drainage systems decrease the variability of the chest tube management in the clinical practice and help decrease the need of provocative clamping maneuvers.
- Both digital and analog drainage systems have been used for modeling the risk of postoperative air leak.
- Despite the need for a consensus to establish the upper limit of daily drainage, 450 mL/24 h of non-chylous clear fluid can be considered safe for chest tube removal.

INTRODUCTION: HOW TO REMOVE A CHEST TUBE

Once a chest tube has been inserted, the most appropriate time for pulling it out is usually a matter of discussion because no sound evidence is available to construct evidence-based guidelines. Usually, chest tube withdrawal policies are dictated by personal preferences and experience, influencing quite variable lengths of stay for the same procedures.

The ideal respiratory phase (end of inspiration or expiration) for removing chest drainages is also debatable. From a physiologic point of view, at the end of expiration the difference between atmospheric and pleural pressures is at its minimum, decreasing the possibility of inadvertent airflow into the pleural space when pulling out pleural tubes. However, at the end of inspiration, lungs are fully expanded and no space between parietal and visceral pleura is left, and that could have also

a beneficial effect. Bell and colleagues[1] designed a prospective randomized study including only trauma subjects. In their study, no differences were found between the 2 different approaches in terms of recurrent pneumothorax and no factors were identified that could adversely influence outcome. The overall rate of recurrent pneumothorax was 7%, and only 3% required chest tube reinsertion. More recently, Cerfolio and colleagues[2] conducted another randomized trial using digital air leak meters that included only lung resection subjects. They found that removal of chest tubes at the end of inspiration produced more recurrent pneumothorax. In fact, the trial was stopped due to significant difference in non-clinically symptomatic pneumothorax at interim analysis. In another study, French and colleagues[3] reviewed all the information about this issue and concluded that tube withdrawal at expiration or inspiration is not crucial as long as a Valsalva maneuver is continued during the procedure.

Conflicts of Interest: The authors have no conflicts of interest to declare.
General Thoracic Surgery Service, University Hospital of Salamanca, Salamanca, Spain
* Corresponding author. Paseo de San Vicente 58-182, Salamanca 37007, Spain.
E-mail address: nuria.novoa@usal.es

Based on this data, the authors recommend that chest tube withdrawal takes place at the end of full expiration during a Valsalva maneuver.

DOES THE PATIENT HAVE AN AIR LEAK?

Postoperative air leak is a common clinical problem after lung surgery. It is dramatically influenced by the quality of the operated lung parenchyma. Because the occurrence of emphysema increases with age and surgeons are currently operating on older patients,[4] the prevalence of the complication is expected to increase despite technical improvements. Postoperative air leak is considered an adverse postoperative event when patient discharge is consequently delayed or outpatient clinic checkups are needed after the patient is discharged with a chest tube in place. Currently, prolonged air leak (PAL) is defined as when a postoperative air leak persists after 5 days, which it is the standard hospital stay for lobectomy in many centers.[5,6] PAL is a source of more serious complications[7] and expenses.[5] In the European Society of Thoracic Surgeons Database 2015 annual report,[4] which included more than 62,000 lung resection procedures, the overall prevalence of PAL was 7.2%, ranging from 3.4% in wedge resection to 23.3% in lung volume reduction procedure. For lobectomy, the reported rate was 8.6%, and 6.7% in cases of segmentectomy.

The presence of air leak is, of course, a contraindication for chest tube withdrawal and should be accurately diagnosed. The thoracic drainage is intended to maintain intrapleural negative pressures and restore the normal intrapleural equilibrium through a water seal that acts as a unidirectional valve system. In conventional systems, the swing of the water column identifies the different phases of the respiratory cycle[8] and the bubbling is evidence of consistent air leak from the lung surface.

In some situations, the diagnosis of air leakage from the parenchyma can be more difficult. First is when the patients have nonconsistent air leak. Intermittent or recurrent air leaks can frequently occur after lung resection with moderate-to-severe chronic obstructive pulmonary disease (COPD).[9] In those cases, keeping the chest tube in place during the first 24 hours after lung resection, even in the absence of air leak, can be adopted as a precaution.

Another difficult situation appears when bubbling at the end of expiration is combined with a high differential pleural pressure (20 cm H_2O). Then, it is necessary to distinguish between an active air leak and a pleural space effect. In this situation, the water seal column moves widely between the inspiratory and the expiratory phase, provoking a final bubbling. Using analogic water seal drainages distinguishing which is the origin of the bubbling is not easy. This problem has been resolved using digital devices capable of recording continuous pressure changes. As Marasco and colleagues[10] demonstrated, a real air leak produces an increased expiratory pressure (-1 to $+4$cm H_2O). On the other hand, space effects are characterized by a high differential pleural pressure due to a lower mean inspiratory pressure (-17 to -30 cm H_2O). Furthermore, an active air leak is more often associated with a continuous transpleural airflow (>20 mL/min) unlike a pleural space effect (<10 mL/min). In this series no subject identify as having a pleural space effect had complications after 24 hours of provocative clamping.

In the analog systems, recording is not available; therefore, the decision to remove the tube is usually made at bedside after asking the patient to perform some respiratory maneuvers. In these settings, the decision process has some inherent subjectivity. This point was clearly demonstrated in a prospective controlled study.[11] The investigators showed that the agreement between 2 senior surgeons on the decision of pulling out chest tubes during morning rounds was very low (0.37%). The disagreement was basically due to the air leak evaluation. The other major objective of that investigation was to evaluate whether the use of an electronic device to measure postoperative air leak decreased this disagreement. The study found that Kappa coefficient rose to 0.88 using the digital system.

Since the introduction of digital air leak meters, the posted question should probably be modified to, "Does the patient have a clinically relevant air leak?" Because the electronic drainage system is able to quantify air leaks and intrathoracic pressures, it contributes objective measures for better and more homogeneous chest tube management.[11] In 2006, Anegg and colleagues[12] performed an interesting study validating the first digital postoperative chest tube airflow meter. The objective of their study was quantifying air leaks using a new digital tool to define the most appropriate moment for the chest tube removal. They recorded the airflow using under different suction settings and after normal breathing, deep breath, cough, and breathing against the resistance of a flutter valve. Probably the most interesting finding was that 15% of the subjects without visual presence of air leak still had a measurable air loss that lasted up to 7 days. They set up the cut-off point for chest tube withdrawal below 20 mL/min during normal breathing on a Heimlich valve because this amount of air was considered normal due to shifts in the measuring system itself.

Based on this previous experience, Brunelli and colleagues[13] developed a new protocol for chest tube management using a new electronic pleural drainage capable of continuous recording of air leakage and intrapleural pressures measurement. For decision purposes, they used the means of the measures recorded during the previous 6 hours. In 62% of the subjects (5/8) with air leak lower than 15 mL/min, provocative clamping was successful. That cutoff value deserves external validation. Recently, a multicenter Canadian group[14] published the results of a prospective randomized trial designed for evaluating the impact of the digital drainage versus the analog system after lung resection on time to chest tube removal and length of stay. Their protocol allowed chest tube withdrawal at the water seal group when no bubbling was present. At the digital drainage group, chest tube removal was considered safe when air leak was equal to or less than 40 mL/min under negative pressure (>8 mm Hg) or equal to or less than 20 mL/min when no suction was applied (<8 mm Hg), at least, during the previous 12 hours. In the final analysis, no statistical differences were found in terms of complications between groups although subjects in the analogic arm had more chest tube reinsertions for worsening pneumothorax or subcutaneous emphysema.

IS PROVOCATIVE CLAMPING STILL NEEDED BEFORE CHEST TUBE REMOVAL?

There is no consensus on the actual benefits of digital compared with analogic drainage systems after lung resection. In their prospective randomized study, Gilbert and colleagues[14] showed that digital drainage systems significantly decreased the number of clamping attempts. As previously mentioned,[10] no provocative clamping test is necessary provided a digital continuous recording drainage device is used that shows that the patient is presenting with no air leak or changes in pleural pressures, suggesting a pleural space effect.

What about analog systems? This issue has not been specifically addressed by any study, yet many groups maintain this practice. Probably, this practice has a role in the management of some difficult or high-risk patients (eg, after a surgical pulmonary biopsy in the context of advanced interstitial disease). Instead, as Cerfolio and colleagues[15] posted, PAL can be treated in an outpatient basis using portable devices,[16] decreasing the length of hospital stay and allowing for safe patient discharge.

IS IT POSSIBLE TO PREDICT THE OCCURRENCE OF PROLONGED AIR LEAK?

Multiple factors are known to be linked to the risk of PAL. Probably, low forced expiratory volume in 1 second (FEV_1) and diffuse emphysema are the most important ones, although important pleural adhesions, inflammatory chronic disease, and upper lobe lobectomy have also been suggested to have important roles.[17] Recently, a nationwide retrospective study assessing this problem was released.[18] After the analysis of more than 24,000 subjects, the investigators developed a predictive model based on gender, body mass index, dyspnea score, presence or absence of pleural adhesions, type of lung resection, and location of the lung to be removed. The model was validated in an external cohort of 6000 subjects showing a concordance index (C-index) of 0.71 (95% CI 0.70–0.72) and a calibration slope of 0.99. Note that a variable as important as FEV_1 had to be excluded from the analysis due to a large number of missing data. The investigators used the dyspnea score to replace FEV_1 and other pulmonary function parameters that were missing in the dataset. On the other hand, the model is robust enough as the high confidence intervals reveal. In 2015, another French group[19] validated this predictive model in a video-assisted thoracic (VATS) anatomic lung resection population, showing also a good adjustment (C-index: 0.72; 95% CI 0.67–0.77; calibration slope of 1.25 (0.9–1.58), and Hosmer-Lemeshow goodness-of-fit test; $P = .35$).

It was interesting to find that Rivera and colleagues[18] concluded that their model can help identify patients at risk for PAL so that intraoperative preventive maneuvers can be performed and digital drainage can be indicated for quantification of air leak. As previously mentioned, digital devices can add to the clinical management of chest tubes, especially in the agreement between surgeons on the presence or absence of air loss,[10] and to decrease the number of clamping trials.[14] Furthermore, Brunelli and colleagues,[20] using digital devices, described 4 groups with different air leak risks. Those groups were based on the different behavior of the differential pressure and the measured flow. They identified 2 categories with special high risk of PAL: (1) those with a differential pressure greater than 10 cm H_2O and airflow less than 50 mL/min with a 4-fold risk and (2) those with greater than 50 mL/min with a 13-fold increased risk over those with a differential pressure inferior to 10 cm H_2O and less than 50 mL/min of airflow. Nevertheless, in a prospective randomized trial, Gilbert and colleagues[14] found that digital drainages add no advantages to air leak management when compared with water seal analog systems in terms of improvement of the analyzed main outcomes: length of stay and duration of chest tube drainage. Probably, as those investigators discussed, digital pleural technology is at its beginning and future devices will improve safety and efficiency in the management of chest tubes. Meanwhile, water seal devices can also help in predicting PAL. Rodriguez and colleagues[21] constructed a simple prediction model for PAL using the preoperative PAL score described previously[22] and the airflow measured at the water seal chamber of an analog drainage. This simple prospective model showed a good predictive capacity reaching a C-index of 0.83 (95% CI 0.73–0.93).

DAILY PLEURAL DRAINAGE, A SAFE THRESHOLD FOR CHEST TUBE REMOVAL

Air leak is not the only limit to the possibility of chest tube removal, the quality and the amount of fluid are also crucial. Probably, the maximum daily pleural output is the parameter with the highest variability between surgeons (outputs ranging between 200 and 500 mL/24 h are admitted). Again, no evidence supports most of the current practices and agreement is necessary to establish an upper volume limit for a safe and efficient procedure. Of course, it is not arguable that the presence of chylous, blood, or purulent fluid are contraindications for chest tube removal.

Under physiologic conditions, daily pleural output is estimated to be around 350 to 400 mL of hypo-oncotic clear liquid. Normal resorption is accomplished both at the parietal and visceral pleura. This is a very efficient mechanism because a 10-fold increase in pleural fluid results in a 15% increase in pleural liquid volume.[23] Injury to the pleura produces an imbalance between normal filtration and resorption. Furthermore, it alters the normal composition of the pleural fluid, increasing the amount of protein in it. However, this change in composition returns to almost normal values very quickly. According to Olgac and colleagues,[24] the blood protein ratio (PrRPI/B) decreases below 0.5, the cut-off value for exudates, in most patients by the second postoperative day and remains low for the subsequent days if no complication occurs. This fact, together with the high absorption capacity of the pleura, allows chest tubes removal even in the presence of larger amount of daily fluid because it can be anticipated. In their prospective study, in the absence of air leak, subjects in the control group had the chest tube withdrawn if the daily drainage was equal to or less than 250 mL

and subjects in the case group had the chest tube removed when PrRPI/B was equal or less than 0.5, regardless of its daily draining amount. No subject required a new chest tube insertion and no further hospital admission for this cause took place. Further studies are necessary to validate these findings. To reproduce the study, it is important to keep in mind that pleural fluid samples should be taken from the chest tubes, not from the collection system, because it has been shown that the diagnostic values of samples taken from the collection bottles have certain variability regarding the amount of proteins and other parameters.[25]

In 2008, Cerfolio and Bryant[26] reported the results of a retrospective study of more than 1900 subjects in whom a chest tube was removed with up to 450 mL/24 h and described the reasons for readmission if it ever occurred. No differences were found between those subjects discharged after removing the chest tube with high output compared with those with daily output equal to or less than 250 mL/24 h. Only 0.55% of the subjects were readmitted due to a recurrent symptomatic effusion, leading to the conclusion that chest tubes can be safely withdrawn with daily outputs up to 450 mL/24 h. Nevertheless, Grodzki[27] could not reproduce these results, opening the door for controversy. Recently[28] chest tube removal after VATS lobectomy was proposed with drainages up to 500 mL/24 h. The investigators of this study recorded only 2.8% of subjects necessitating retreatment for symptomatic pleural effusion after chest drainage removal.

Different types of lobectomy seem to have different postoperative fluid output. In this observational study,[29] higher fluid outputs were reported after lower lobectomy compared with upper ones; the right lower lobectomy the one registered the highest amount. Both right and left upper lobectomies showed equal amount of fluid drainage losses. This finding indicates that lower lobectomy damage is the most important area of the pleura responsible for fluid resorption that is located at the basal part of the pleural space.[23] Again, these findings show a wide amount of opportunities for investigation around chest tube removal after different lung resections.

Finally, high pleural output drainage seems to be also predictable. Age (≥70 years), lower lobectomy, and the presence of COPD were the independent variables introduced in the aggregate classification model.[30] According to the total calculated score, subjects were ordered in classes of incremental risk. The cut-off point for chest tube removal in this prospective study was 400 mL/24 h. For COPD patients older than 70 years undergoing right lower lobectomy, the risk of developing a large pleural effusion is 39%. Although the authors recommend using this risk score for introducing preventive interventions and careful drainage withdrawal during the postoperative period, external validation of these results would be advisable.

REFERENCES

1. Bell RL, Ovadia P, Abdullah F, et al. Chest tube removal: End-inspiration or End-expiration? J Trauma 2001;50: 674–7.

2. Cerfolio RJ, Bryant AS, Skylizard L, et al. Optimal technique for the removal of chest tubes after pulmonary resection. J Thorac Cardiovasc Surg 2013; 145:1535–9.

3. French DG, Dilena M, LaPlante S, et al. Optimizing postoperative care protocols in thoracic surgery: best evidence and new technology. J Thorac Dis 2016;8(Suppl 1):S3–11.

4. Database report Silver Book 2015. p. 30, 37. Available at: http://www.ests.org/_userfiles/pages/files/ESTS%20201Silver_Book_FULL_PEF.pdf. Accessed February 15, 2016.

5. Varela G, Jiménez MF, Novoa N, et al. Estimating hospital costs attributable to prolonged air leak in pulmonary lobectomy. Eur J Cardiothorac Surg 2005;27:329–33.

6. Pompili C, Miserocchi G. Air leak after lung resection: pathophysiology and patients' implications. J Thorac Dis 2016;8(Suppl 1):S46–54.

7. Brunelli A, Xiumé F, Al Refai M, et al. Air leaks after lobectomy increase the risk of empyema but not of cardiopulmonary complications: a case-matched analysis. Chest 2006;130:1150–6.

8. Brunelli A, Beretta E, Cassivi SD, et al. Consensus definitions to promote an evidence-based approach to management of the pleural space. A collaborative proposal by ESTS, AATS, STS and GTSC. Eur J Cardiothorac Surg 2011;40:291–7.

9. Pompili C, Salati M, Refai M, et al. Recurrent air leak soon after pulmonary lobectomy: an analysis based on an electronic airflow evaluation†. Eur J Cardiothorac Surg 2016;49:1091–4.

10. Marasco RD, Giudice G, Lequaglie C. How to distinguish an active air leak from a pleural space effect. Asian Cardiovasc Thorac Ann 2012;20:682–8.

11. Varela G, Jiménez MF, Novoa N, et al. Postoperative chest tube management: measuring air leak using an electronic device decreases variability in the clinical practice. Eur J Cardiothorac Surg 2009;35: 28–31.

12. Anegg U, Lindnmann J, Matzi V, et al. AIRFIX®: the first digital postoperative chest tube airflowmetry—a novel method to quantify air leakage after lung resection. Eur J Cardiothorac Surg 2006;29:867–72.

13. Brunelli A, Salati M, Refai M, et al. Evaluation of a new chest tube removal protocol using digital air leak monitoring after lobectomy: a prospective randomised trial. Eur J Cardiothorac Surg 2010;37: 56–60.

14. Gilbert S, McGuire AL, Maghera S, et al. Randomized trial of digital versus analog pleural drainage in patients with or without a pulmonary air leak after lung resection. J Thorac Cardiovasc Surg 2015;150: 1243–9.

15. Cerfolio RJ, Minnich DJ, Bryant AS. The removal of chest tubes despite an air leak or a pneumothorax. Ann Thorac Surg 2009;87:1690–6.

16. Varela G, Jiménez MF, Novoa N. Portable chest drainage systems and outpatient chest tube management. Thorac Surg Clin 2010;20:421–6.

17. Mueller MR, Marzluf BA. The anticipation and management of air leaks and residual spaces post lung resection. J Thorac Dis 2014;6:271–84.

18. Rivera C, Bernard A, Falcoz PE, et al. Characterization and prediction of prolonged air leak after pulmonary resection: a nationwide study setting up the index of prolonged air leak. Ann Thorac Surg 2011;92:1062–8.

19. Orsini B, Baste JM, Gossot D, et al. Index of prolonged air leak score validation in case of video-assisted thoracoscopic surgery anatomical lung resection: results of a nationwide study based on the French national thoracic database, EPITHOR. Eur J Cardiothorac Surg 2015;48:608–11.

20. Brunelli A, Cassivi SD, Salati M, et al. Digital measurements of air leak flow and intrapleural pressures in the immediate postoperative period predict risk of prolonged air leak after pulmonary lobectomy. Eur J Cardiothorac Surg 2011;39:584–8.

21. Rodriguez M, Jiménez MF, Hernández MT, et al. Usefulness of conventional pleural drainage systems to predict the occurrence of prolonged air leak after anatomical pulmonary resection. Eur J Cardiothorac Surg 2015;48:612–5.

22. Brunelli A, Varela G, Refai M, et al. A scoring system to predict the risk of prolonged air leak after lobectomy. Ann Thorac Surg 2010;90:204–9.

23. Miserocchi G. Physiology and pathophysiology of pleural fluid turnover. Eur Respir J 1997;10: 219–25.

24. Olgac G, Casgun T, Vayvada M, et al. Low protein content of drainage fluid is a good predictor for earlier chest tube removal after lobectomy. Interact Cardiovasc Thorac Surg 2014;19:650–5.

25. Reed RM, Eberlein M, Netzer G, et al. Diagnostic value of pleural fluid obtained from a chest tube collection system. Lung 2015;193:141–6.

26. Cerfolio RJ, Bryant AS. Results of a prospective algorithm to remove chest tubes after pulmonary resection with high output. J Thorac Cardiovasc Surg 2008;135:269–73.

27. Grodzki T. Prospective algorithm to remove chest tubes after pulmonary resection with high output-is it valid everywhere? J Thorac Cardiovasc Surg 2008;136:536.

28. Bjerregaard LS, Jensen K, Petersen RH, et al. Early chest tube removal after video-assisted thoracic surgery lobectomy with serous fluid production up to 500 ml/day. Eur J Cardiothorac Surg 2014;45:241–6.

29. Kouritas VK, Zissis C, Bellenis I. Variation of the postoperative fluid drainage according to the type of lobectomy. Interact Cardiovasc Thorac Surg 2013;16:437–40.

30. Hristova R, Pompili C, Begum S, et al. An aggregate score to predict the risk of large pleural effusion after pulmonary lobectomy. Eur J Cardiothorac Surg 2015;48:72–6.

Indwelling Pleural Catheters
A Clinical Option in Trapped Lung

Luca Bertolaccini, MD, PhD[a],*, Andrea Viti, MD, PhD[a],
Simona Paiano, MD[b], Carlo Pomari, MD[b],
Luca Rosario Assante, MD[b], Alberto Terzi, MD[a]

KEYWORDS

• Indwelling pleural catheter • Lung cancer • Malignant pleural effusion • Palliative treatments

KEY POINTS

- Malignant pleural effusion (MPE) is a form of advanced cancer and is associated with short-term median survival.
- Ideal treatment of MPE should achieve effective long-term symptom relief, minimize hospitalization, and reduce adverse effects.
- Indwelling pleural catheter (IPC) is a useful option for the management of MPE.
- IPC offers advantages over pleurodesis in patients unfit for pleurodesis and controls symptoms in patients with trapped lung.
- IPC can be used in patients with poor performance status or with high surgical risk and short life expectancy.

INTRODUCTION

MPE is a complication of almost any site of primary cancer as well as primary tumors of the pleura. The most common presenting symptoms of MPE are dyspnea, cough, and chest pain. All these symptoms have a real impact on quality of life (QOL). On the other hand, from an oncological point of view, MPE always represents a form of advanced cancer and is associated with a short-term median survival that varies according to the primary tumor site.[1] The palliation of MPE can be performed with a surgical approach through VATS under general anesthesia. In patients unfit for general anesthesia, awake pleuroscopy represents an alternative for pleurodesis because it is usually performed under conscious sedation and local anesthesia alone. Also, sclerosing agents can be administered at the bedside through a chest tube. To date, randomized trials have failed to show the superiority of VATS/pleuroscopy versus bedside chest tube approaches, when pleurodesis is the primary study endpoint. Nevertheless, many physicians assume thoracoscopic/pleuroscopic ways are superior based on their personal experience and secondary outcome analyses reported in the literature. Nowadays, talc is widely regarded as the best agent for pleurodesis. Many agents display a different form of efficacy as pleurodesis agents (**Table 1**).[1,2] For VATS or pleuroscopic procedures, patients with MPE frequently require hospitalization. Nevertheless, for these patients, the real priority is to minimize the days spent at the hospital, thereby

Disclosure Statement: The authors have nothing to disclosure.
[a] Thoracic Surgery Unit, Sacro Cuore Don Calabria Research Hospital – Cancer Care Center, Via Don Angelo Sempreboni 5, Negrar, Verona 37024, Italy; [b] Thoracic Endoscopy Unit, Sacro Cuore Don Calabria Research Hospital – Cancer Care Center, Via Don Angelo Sempreboni 5, Negrar, Verona 37024, Italy
* Corresponding author.
E-mail address: luca.bertolaccini@gmail.com

Thorac Surg Clin 27 (2017) 47–55
http://dx.doi.org/10.1016/j.thorsurg.2016.08.008
1547-4127/17/© 2016 Elsevier Inc. All rights reserved.

Table 1
The rate of success of chemical pleurodesis

Pleurodesis Agent	Pleurodesis (%)	Reference
Talc slurry (2–5 g)	90	[36]
Talc poudrage (2–5 g)	93.4	[37]
Tetracycline (1–1.5 g)	67	[37]
Others	>50	[38]

Data from Simoff MJ, Lally B, Slade MG, et al. Symptom management in patients with lung cancer: diagnosis and management of lung cancer, 3rd ed: American College of Chest Physicians evidence-based clinical practice guidelines. Chest 2013;143(5 Suppl):e455S–97S.

allowing them back home as soon as possible. The ideal treatment of MPE should include adequate and enduring relief from symptoms (in particular dyspnea), minimize hospitalization, and reduce adverse effects.[3] The IPC is increasingly used for the management of MPE[4] and is preferred for patients with a trapped lung or failed pleurodesis (**Table 2**).[5]

THERAPEUTIC OPTIONS
When Can Patients Be Proposed Indwelling Pleural Catheter Placement?

IPCs are typically inserted on an outpatient basis under local anesthesia followed by drainage at home performed by trained family members or dedicated home care providers.[6] IPC aims to intermittently drain the MPE to maintain an adequate lung expansion without a attempt at causing pleurodesis. With IPC alone, approximately half of patients eventually achieve pleurodesis. IPC is effective in controlling symptoms not only in MPE but also in patients with trapped lung (**Table 3**).[7] Patients with poor performance status or high surgical risk should be considered for IPC placement because patients with longer survival should preferentially be offered pleurodesis rather than IPC.[8] In patients with extremely low survival (days or few weeks), the optimal treatment consists of thoracentesis plus systemic administration of opioids.[1] IPC could be used in patients whose expected survival is longer with excellent outcomes. IPC could also be used during systemic chemotherapy.[9] IPC could be placed in patients with underlying hematologic malignancy and significant immunosuppression because a similar overall infection rate to another procedure has been reported in previous studies.[10] Not last, IPC seems a safe and effective treatment of MPE in advanced pediatric cancer, achieving the relief of symptoms and shortening hospitalization.[11]

The World Market of Indwelling Pleural Catheters

The first report in the literature of a patient sent home with an IPC was in 1986 when a Tenckhoff catheter was placed with drainage at the patient's home twice a week. The Copernican revolution in MPE management was the approval of the PleurX catheter (Denver Biomedical, Golden, Colorado) in

Table 2
The options of treatment of malignant pleural effusion

Option of Treatment	Indication	Notes
Repetitive thoracentesis	Recurrent effusion in patients with poor performance status Short expected survival	High recurrence rate Complications: pneumothorax, empyema
Talc slurry	Symptomatic recurrent large effusion	Alternative to pleurodesis via pleuroscopy Not available in trapped lung
Talc poudrage	Symptomatic recurrent large effusion	Not available in trapped lung
Indwelling pleural catheter	Symptomatic recurrent effusion in patients with poor performance status Trapped lung Failed pleurodesis in patient with good health and long survival	Costs Catheter obstructions Catheter tract metastasis (?)

Data from Simoff MJ, Lally B, Slade MG, et al. Symptom management in patients with lung cancer: diagnosis and management of lung cancer, 3rd ed: American College of Chest Physicians evidence-based clinical practice guidelines. Chest 2013;143(5 Suppl):e455S–97S.

Table 3
The quality-of-life (QOL) and dyspnea scores of indwelling pleural catheter and pleurodesis

	Score Type	Significantly Improved (%)	Unchanged or Deteriorated (%)
QOL	IPC	93.3	6.7
	pleurodesis	50	50
Dyspnea	IPC	93.3	6.7
	pleurodesis	78.6	21.4

Data from Fysh ET, Waterer GW, Kendall PA, et al. Indwelling pleural catheters reduce inpatient days over pleurodesis for malignant pleural effusion. Chest 2012;142(2):394–400.

1997 by the Food and Drug Administration for use as IPC to drain the recurrent MPE intermittently.[12] After this approval, the use of IPC has been enrolled in the armamentarium of management of MPE. A competitor is the Aspira pleural drainage system (Bard Access Systems, Salt Lake City, Utah); the design is similar to PleurX, but the main difference is that instead of using vacuum bottles for pleural drainage, the Aspira catheter uses a manual pump. Another catheter manufacturer is Rocket Medical (Washington, Tyne & Wear, United Kingdom) with a design similar to the PleurX catheter.[13] From 2014, the Relief system is being produced and commercialized (Med-Italia Biomedica, Genoa, Italy). This device is also similar to PleurX (**Fig. 1**).[14]

Brief Overview of the Surgical Technique of Indwelling Pleural Catheter Placement

Several methods of placement of the IPC have been described in the literature. This article outlines the methods of placement as reported elsewhere.[13,14] Ultrasonography allows a surgeon to locate MPE and confirm the site of insertion. The entry site and the counter-incision are marked with an indelible marker (**Fig. 2**). After preprocedural planning, the skin is cleansed with an antiseptic solution over an extended surface around the IPC insert sites as well as along the entirety of the tunnel. Lidocaine 2%, 20 mL, is used as local anesthesia to inoculate the skin and the soft tissues up to the level of the parietal pleura and along the length of the tunnel. On the track identified during the initial anesthesia, a guide needle is then advanced while aspirating (**Fig. 3**). Once pleural fluid is seen in the syringe, the guide wire is passed through the needle into the pleural space, and then the needle is removed (**Fig. 4**). Two incisions are made at the entry site (pleural entry site) and exit sites (catheter from the skin) (**Fig. 5**). The authors suggest shortening the skin incision in the planned exit site to allow the precise exit of the catheter from the skin, minimizing the possible risk of IPC dislocation. The IPC is then

passed through the skin exit site toward the pleural entry site. This maneuver is allowed by the tunneling tool, generally provided with the catheter by the manufacturer (**Fig. 6**). After that, the dilator device is passed over the guide wire to create the route for the introducer (**Fig. 7**). Once entering the pleura, the dilator and the guide wire are removed, and the IPC is rapidly advanced through the peel-away (Med-Italia Biomedica, Genoa, Italy) introducer to minimize the flow of air into the pleural space (**Fig. 8**). Once the entire catheter is advanced through the sheath, it is peeled apart and removed (**Fig. 9**). The incision is closed, and the catheter is secured to the skin with a suture

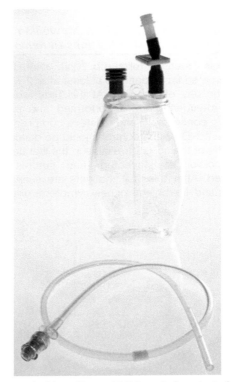

Fig. 1. Relief is a 65-cm, 15.5-French fenestrated silicone catheter. (*Courtesy of* Med-Italia Biomedica Genoa, Italy; with permission.)

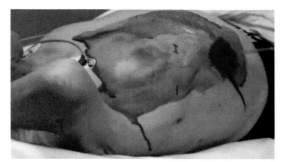

Fig. 2. The entry site and the counter-incision are marked with an indelible marker.

material. Once the IPC is secured, the pleural space is drained. The drainage line is connected to the 1-way valve at the end of the IPC. Pleural fluid is removed until the patient developed symptoms, such as cough, pain, or dyspnea. The drainage system is then disconnected, and the plastic valve cap provided is secured onto the valve. A foamy drain sponge is placed over the IPC to prevent decubitus. A chest radiograph is performed after catheter insertion to ensure the adequate placement and the absence of immediate complications. Once a physician reviews the roentgenogram, the patient can be discharged home.[13,14]

Management at Home of the Indwelling Pleural Catheter and Indications to Removal

A single routine follow-up visit should be programmed for all patients at least after 2 weeks after the day of insertion. At this time, another chest roentgenogram is performed and symptoms, concerns, and late complications addressed. Dyspnea control should be described with one of the scales available in the literature.[15] The incision is inspected, and sutures are removed. After this visit, patients are seen only on demand, if problems or new symptoms develop

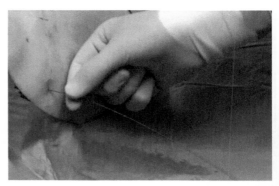

Fig. 4. The guide wire is passed through the needle into the pleural space.

or if IPC removal is indicated. Follow-up and support by well-trained district nurses are scheduled on an outpatient basis with at least a weekly visit.[7] A weekly fluid evacuation is recommended, until less than 500 mL is obtained and, in this case, more time should elapse the visits between evacuations. Mainly, a complete successful pleurodesis is defined as long-term symptom relief, with the absence of fluid accumulation on the chest radiograph whereas a successful partial pleurodesis indicates the diminution of dyspnea related to effusion, with an only partial accumulation of MPE, without the need for further thoracentesis. When no drainage takes place for 1 month, and a chest roentgenogram shows no significant MPE, the possible removal under local anesthesia can be offered to the patient.[14] Several factors should be observed during the placement process, to avoid break of the IPC during the removal.

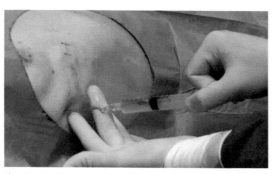

Fig. 3. On the track identified during the initial anesthesia, a guide needle is then advanced while aspirating.

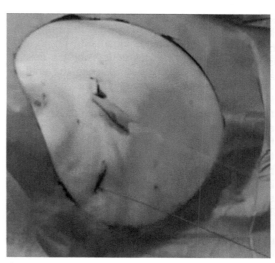

Fig. 5. Two incisions made at the pleural entry site and the exit sites of catheter from the skin.

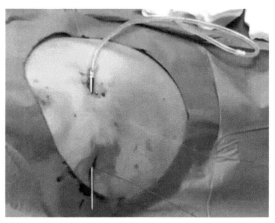

Fig. 6. The IPC is passed through the skin exit site toward the pleural entry site.

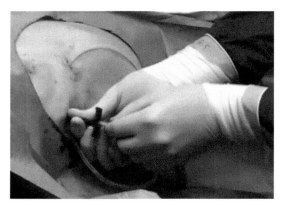

Fig. 8. The IPC is advanced through the peel-away introducer.

The location of the polyester cuff within 1 cm of the tunnel entry site is crucial to facilitate the IPC removal; more distant placement of the IPC cuff within the tunnel increases the risk of weakening the catheter. The subcutaneous tunnelization ideally should be less than 5 cm because longer subcutaneous tracts may result in IPC fenestrations outside the pleural cavity, causing the tissue ingrowths and impending the removal procedure.[16]

CLINICAL OUTCOMES
Benefits in Trapped Lung

Proper pulmonary re-expansion before pleurodesis should be demonstrated because a trapped lung is considered a contraindication to VATS and pleuroscopy: pleurodesis can be achieved only in patients whose lung displays a full re-expansion after a thoracentesis.[6] Nevertheless, more than half of MPE patients have nonexpandable trapped lungs not suitable for talc pleurodesis.[17] IPC, however, can be used in this cohort of patients, bringing about an improvement in

dyspnea and QOL that is comparable to talc pleurodesis.[18] As discussed previously, lung re-expansion must be considered when planning for pleurodesis. In patients with trapped lungs, IPC remains one of the unique options for palliation of dyspnea related to recurrent MPE.

Hospitalization

VATS or pleuroscopy requires hospitalization with a median hospital length of stay of 4 to 5 days, whereas IPC is often inserted as 1-day surgical procedure.[19] In a nonrandomized trial, patients treated with IPC spent significantly fewer days in the hospital (for any causes) from procedure to death than from pleurodesis and these benefits influence the treatment choice in MPE.[18]

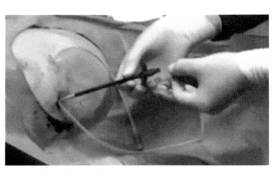

Fig. 7. The dilator device is passed over the guide wire to create the route for the introducer.

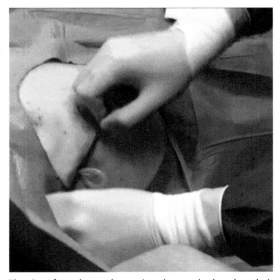

Fig. 9. After the catheter is advanced, the sheath is peeled apart and removed.

Pleurodesis

Pleurodesis provokes intense pleural and systemic inflammation with pain and fever sometimes severe. Talc pleurodesis can cause hypoxemia and, in severe cases, acute respiratory failure.[20] The IPC avoids these disadvantages and could be used in frail patients.[18] Pleurodesis is not the primary endpoint of IPC treatment; nevertheless, an overall spontaneous pleurodesis rate of 45% was reported,[12] but when limiting the inclusion criteria to patients who may have been candidates for pleurodesis, pleurodesis rates climb to 70%.[21] IPC-related pleurodesis has been reported between 29 and 59 days after placement.[1] The IPC placement allows the safe and efficient palliation of MPE in an outpatient setting. Management of symptoms as an outpatient allows patients to maintain control over their lives and minimizes the time the spent in the hospital. A systematic review reported symptom improvement in 95.6% of patients and spontaneous pleurodesis in 45.6%; the IPC was removed in 47.1% of those patients. The recurrence of the effusion after the catheter removal is less than than 8%.[12] Hybrid approaches using IPC insertion at the same time of pleuroscopic talc pleurodesis have been proposed.[22] Hybrid approaches reduce the number of days in the hospital after thoracoscopy as well as lessen the time that a patient maintains the IPC. Nevertheless, additional studies are still required.[23] At this time, there are no results from the Australasian Malignant Pleural Effusion trial, a multicenter, randomized trial designed to compare the IPC with talc pleurodesis. The primary endpoint evaluated is the total number of days spent in the hospital from the insertion procedure to death whereas secondary endpoints include hospital days specific to MPE management, adverse events, and self-reported symptom and QOL scores.[4] In a study of predictors of the likelihood of receiving pleurodesis with IPC, patients with MPE of lower pleural fluid pH and large sizes were significantly more likely to receive definitive therapy.[22] Several investigators have suggested that low pleural pH signifies greater disease burden and metabolic activities in the pleural space, which may determine the likelihood and rapidity of accumulation of MPE.[24] Furthermore, prospective studies are needed to establish whether pleural pH improves patient selection and, if so, what is the best cutoff value.[25] In another study, the possible measurement of QOL-adjusted survival after IPC placement for MPE found that IPC was associated with substantial improvements in dyspnea but modest improvements in utility. Patients who had more

dyspnea at baseline and who were able to receive treatment after IPC placement had the greatest increase in efficiency. As such, the marginal benefit of leaving IPC for a long time to prevent recurrence may be warranted only in select patients, depending on how long the IPC has been in place and how much drainage there is. The focus should be on using patient-centered outcomes and the proper use of time-to-event analysis rather than radiographic outcomes and incidence proportions.[26] The Second Therapeutic Intervention in Malignant Effusion, an unblinded randomized controlled trial comparing IPC and talc pleurodesis, demonstrates that both strategies are highly effective treatments for relieving dyspnea and shows that there was no significant difference in the clinically relevant outcome measures of chest pain and QOL between these treatments. Apparently, IPC cannot be advocated as a superior treatment to talc pleurodesis for palliation of symptoms. Other factors, however, such as hospital length of stay, adverse events, and the inconvenience of ongoing drainage, may be significant factors in patient's and physician's choice of initial treatment modality in MPE. The overall cost of these treatments will be an important factor in determining which treatments are offered in the future.[20]

COMPLICATIONS AND CONCERNS
The Nightmare of Indwelling Pleural Catheter: The Costs

The cost of an IPC may be an issue due to the expense of the device and the single-use vacuum bottles.[19] IPC management causes some direct (eg, drainage kits and personnel support for drainage assistance) and indirect (eg, management of possible IPC complications costs) expenses. Nevertheless, several factors significantly affect the overall cost of IPC management, such as IPC insertion (inpatient vs outpatient), duration of IPC in situ (function of survival and rates of spontaneous pleurodesis), complication rates, drainage regimes and frequency (daily vs symptom-guided), and not least the need for additional community support (family member vs nurse-assisted drainage). These factors could vary widely in individual patients and make a difficult cost analysis of IPC. In general, the costs of IPC treatment increase, because the IPC is in situ for longer, with greater requirements for drainage consumables.[27] Most studies on IPC cost analysis are retrospective and used the indirect comparisons with conventional treatments. IPC was cost-effective in patients with very short (weeks) survival.[28] Data collected from the Second Therapeutic Intervention in Malignant Effusion randomized controlled study found no significant difference in the overall cost of IPC versus talc pleurodesis.[29] The prices of items vary among countries.[18] A cost-effectiveness decision model of IPC versus bedside pleurodesis, repeated thoracentesis, and pleuroscopic talc pleurodesis found IPC superior to the other therapeutic options. These findings, however, were limited to patients with short life expectancy (overall survival <3 months). If the percentage of spontaneous pleurodesis fell or the complication rates increased, the cost-effectiveness of IPC was reduced. Identifying predictors of survival in patients with MPE may be helpful in deciding which management strategy may be best for patients.[29]

Pleural Infection

Bacterial colonization can occur in patients with IPC whose pleural fluid yields positive microbiology, without the clinical manifestation of frank empyema or the typical biochemical profile of infected pleural fluid. Nevertheless, IPC-related pleural infections have generally been reported as mild.[30]

Malfunction

A dense fibrinous tissue around or within the IPC can occasionally cause lumen obstruction, although complete occlusion IPC is uncommon. Flushing with saline may dislodge the occluding materials and could re-establish patency. Blocked IPC in patients with little residual MPE should be removed to prevent infection.[18]

Loculations

Symptomatic pleural loculation is a frequent complication of IPC. When symptomatic loculations develop, the primary aim of palliating dyspnea in patients with an IPC becomes difficult. Often, these patients have limited options. Many have to undergo further invasive procedures (pleural aspirations or removal of the ineffective IPC and replacement by another IPC or chest drain) or are restricted to pharmacologic palliation of their breathlessness. The related hospitalizations as well as the increased risks and costs of additional procedures could be reduced if pleural drainage via the IPC could be re-established successfully by breaking down the pleural loculations.[31]

Indwelling Pleural Catheter Tract Metastasis

Catheter tract metastasis may develop in patients with malignancies besides mesothelioma. The risk of IPC-related catheter tract metastasis may be higher because IPC is often placed for the rest of a patient's life and may, therefore, pose a permanent risk of tumor seeding.[32] As far as mesothelioma is concerned, the benefit of prophylactic irradiation of the tunnelization site remains controversial. The available randomized clinical trials are based on results of small sample sizes with inadequate statistical power; nevertheless, large prospective studies are difficult to realize due to the low incidence of mesothelioma. Based on the available data, the prophylactic irradiation of the intervention tract is not currently justified.[33] On the contrary, in recent study, investigators report the histologic findings of IPC removed from 41 patients with underlying pleural malignancy over a 54-month period. Mesothelioma was the underlying malignancy in a majority of cases. There was no evidence of a direct tumor invasion or growth of cancer cells on the catheter surfaces. The presence of malignant cells was seen within organizing fibrinous tissues in the lumen of 27% of IPC; after that, the IPC material does not support direct tumor growth or invasion even in the setting of high mesothelioma prevalence.[34]

SUMMARY

IPC represents a therapeutic opportunity, and there is still room for improvement. The exact place of IPC in the paradigm of MPE management has yet to be defined. IPC is accepted for treatment of MPE patients in whom pleurodesis has failed or is contraindicated (mainly trapped lungs). Aftercare of IPC is crucial to its efficient and safe employment. IPCs are often inserted (even within one center) by different specialists—surgeons, radiologists, or pulmonologists—but often the infrastructure established to provide community support and close follow-ups is lacking. A dedicated IPC service, already available in selected centers, is recommended. A centralized IPC service allows clinicians to gain expertise and avoid dilution of experience during the active learning phase. The measurement of success of the IPC by pleurodesis rate, often measured by the absence of fluid on roentgenograms, is of small importance. The success of IPC should be defined as no further effusion-related drainage procedure. The priority for most MPE patients is alleviation of dyspnea and optimization of QOL while avoiding hospital admissions and these are the outcomes to research in the future studies.[35] Although international guidelines on MPE treatment now include the use of an IPC as a viable approach, IPC offers advantages over pleurodesis in patients with poor functional status who cannot tolerate pleurodesis or in patients with trapped lungs. Pleurodesis has a higher chance of resolution of an MPE but requires a hospital stay with a more invasive procedure. IPC is an outpatient, less invasive solution but needs prolonged catheter drainages and home care. The relief of symptoms and the QOL improvement can be accomplished with this approach.[1]

REFERENCES

1. Fortin M, Tremblay A. Pleural controversies: indwelling pleural catheter vs. pleurodesis for malignant pleural effusions. J Thorac Dis 2015;7(6):1052–7.
2. Kastelik JA. Management of malignant pleural effusion. Lung 2013;191(2):165–75.
3. Antunes G, Neville E, Duffy J, et al, Pleural Diseases Group, SoCC, British Thoracic Society. BTS guidelines for the management of malignant pleural effusions. Thorax 2003;58(Suppl 2):ii29–38.
4. Fysh ET, Thomas R, Read CA, et al. Protocol of the Australasian malignant pleural effusion (AMPLE) trial: a multicentre randomised study comparing indwelling pleural catheter versus talc pleurodesis. BMJ Open 2014;4(11):e006757.
5. Zarogoulidis K, Zarogoulidis P, Darwiche K, et al. Malignant pleural effusion and algorithm management. J Thorac Dis 2013;5(Suppl 4):S413–9.
6. Chee A, Tremblay A. The use of tunneled pleural catheters in the treatment of pleural effusions. Curr Opin Pulm Med 2011;17(4):237–41.
7. Efthymiou CA, Masudi T, Thorpe JA, et al. Malignant pleural effusion in the presence of trapped lung. Five-year experience of PleurX tunnelled catheters. Interact Cardiovasc Thorac Surg 2009;9(6):961–4.
8. Bibby AC, Gibbs L, Braybrooke JP. Medical and oncological management of malignant mesothelioma. Br J Hosp Med (Lond) 2015;76(7):384–9.
9. Chan Wah Hak C, Sivakumar P, Ahmed L. Safety of indwelling pleural catheter use in patients undergoing chemotherapy: a five-year retrospective evaluation. BMC Pulm Med 2016;16(1):41.
10. Gilbert CR, Lee HJ, Skalski JH, et al. The use of indwelling tunneled pleural catheters for recurrent pleural effusions in patients with hematologic malignancies: a multicenter study. Chest 2015;148(3):752–8.
11. den Hollander BS, Connolly BL, Sung L, et al. Successful use of indwelling tunneled catheters for the management of effusions in children with advanced cancer. Pediatr Blood Cancer 2014;61(6):1007–12.
12. Van Meter ME, McKee KY, Kohlwes RJ. Efficacy and safety of tunneled pleural catheters in adults with malignant pleural effusions: a systematic review. J Gen Intern Med 2011;26(1):70–6.
13. Gillen J, Lau C. Permanent indwelling catheters in the management of pleural effusions. Thorac Surg Clin 2013;23(1):63–71, vi.
14. Bertolaccini L, Viti A, Terzi A. Management of malignant pleural effusions in patients with trapped lung with indwelling pleural catheter: how to do it. J Visualized Surg 2016;2(44).
15. Filosso PL, Sandri A, Felletti G, et al. Preliminary results of a new small-bore percutaneous pleural catheter used for treatment of malignant pleural effusions in ECOG PS 3-4 patients. Eur J Surg Oncol 2011;37(12):1093–8.
16. Grosu HB, Eapen GA, Morice RC, et al. Complications of removal of indwelling pleural catheters. Chest 2012;142(4):1071 [author reply: 1071–2].
17. Ahmed L, Ip H, Rao D, et al. Talc pleurodesis through indwelling pleural catheters for malignant pleural effusions: retrospective case series of a novel clinical pathway. Chest 2014;146(6):e190–4.
18. Lui MM, Thomas R, Lee YC. Complications of indwelling pleural catheter use and their management. BMJ Open Respir Res 2016;3(1):e000123.
19. Bertolaccini L, Viti A, Gorla A, et al. Home-management of malignant pleural effusion with an indwelling pleural catheter: Ten years experience. Eur J Surg Oncol 2012;38(12):1161–4.
20. Davies HE, Mishra EK, Kahan BC, et al. Effect of an indwelling pleural catheter vs chest tube and talc pleurodesis for relieving dyspnea in patients with malignant pleural effusion: the TIME2 randomized controlled trial. JAMA 2012;307(22):2383–9.
21. Tremblay A, Michaud G. Single-center experience with 250 tunnelled pleural catheter insertions for malignant pleural effusion. Chest 2006;129(2):362–8.
22. Reddy C, Ernst A, Lamb C, et al. Rapid pleurodesis for malignant pleural effusions: a pilot study. Chest 2011;139(6):1419–23.
23. Myers R, Michaud G. Tunneled pleural catheters: an update for 2013. Clin Chest Med 2013;34(1):73–80.
24. Rodriguez-Panadero F, Romero-Romero B. Management of malignant pleural effusions. Curr Opin Pulm Med 2011;17(4):269–73.
25. Fysh ET, Bielsa S, Budgeon CA, et al. Predictors of clinical use of pleurodesis and/or indwelling pleural catheter therapy for malignant pleural effusion. Chest 2015;147(6):1629–34.
26. Ost DE, Jimenez CA, Lei X, et al. Quality-adjusted survival following treatment of malignant pleural effusions with indwelling pleural catheters. Chest 2014;145(6):1347–56.
27. Boshuizen RC, Onderwater S, Burgers SJ, et al. The use of indwelling pleural catheters for the management of malignant pleural effusion–direct costs in a Dutch hospital. Respiration 2013;86(3):224–8.
28. Olden AM, Holloway R. Treatment of malignant pleural effusion: PleuRx catheter or talc pleurodesis? A cost-effectiveness analysis. J Palliat Med 2010;13(1):59–65.
29. Penz ED, Mishra EK, Davies HE, et al. Comparing cost of indwelling pleural catheter vs talc

pleurodesis for malignant pleural effusion. Chest 2014;146(4):991–1000.

30. Mekhaiel E, Kashyap R, Mullon JJ, et al. Infections associated with tunnelled indwelling pleural catheters in patients undergoing chemotherapy. J Bronchology Interv Pulmonol 2013;20(4):299–303.

31. Thomas R, Piccolo F, Miller D, et al. Intrapleural fibrinolysis for the treatment of indwelling pleural catheter-related symptomatic loculations: a multicenter observational study. Chest 2015;148(3):746–51.

32. Thomas R, Budgeon CA, Kuok YJ, et al. Catheter tract metastasis associated with indwelling pleural catheters. Chest 2014;146(3):557–62.

33. Bertolaccini L, Viti A, Terzi A. To seed or not to seed: the open question of mesothelioma intervention tract metastases. Chest 2014;146(3):e111.

34. Tobin CL, Thomas R, Chai SM, et al. Histopathology of removed indwelling pleural catheters from patients with malignant pleural diseases. Respirology 2016;21(5):939–42.

35. Lee YC, Fysh ET. Indwelling pleural catheter: changing the paradigm of malignant effusion management. J Thorac Oncol 2011;6(4):655–7.

36. Simoff MJ, Lally B, Slade MG, Goldberg WG, Lee P, Michaud GC, et al. Symptom management in patients with lung cancer: diagnosis and management of lung cancer, 3rd ed: American College of Chest Physicians evidence-based clinical practice guidelines. Chest 2013;143(5 Suppl):e455S–97S.

37. Walker-Renard PB, Vaughan LM, Sahn SA. Chemical pleurodesis for malignant pleural effusions. Ann Intern Med 1994;120(1):56–64.

38. Kennedy L, Rusch VW, Strange C, Ginsberg RJ, Sahn SA. Pleurodesis using talc slurry. Chest 1994;106(2):342–6.

Errors and Complications in Chest Tube Placement

Pier Luigi Filosso, MD, FECTS[a],*, Francesco Guerrera, MD[a], Alberto Sandri, MD[a],
Matteo Roffinella, MD[a], Paolo Solidoro, MD[b], Enrico Ruffini, MD, FECTS[a], Alberto Oliaro, MD[a]

KEYWORDS

- Chest drainage • Placement • Lung • Pleura • Diaphragm • Errors • Complications

KEY POINTS

- Despite many benefits, drain placement is not always a harmless procedure, and potential significant morbidity and mortality may exist.
- According to the guidelines, to reduce the risk of injury of the underlying vascular structures, the drain should be inserted within the so-called "safe triangle," defined as the thoracic area between the anterior edge of the latissimus dorsi muscle, the lateral edge of the pectoralis major muscle, and a line superior to the horizontal level of the nipple with the apex below the axilla.
- Care should be taken when a drain must be placed in a patient with a previous thoracic/cardiac surgery, or in whom a pleurodesis has been previously achieved.
- Potentially, all the intrathoracic organs (especially the lung, the diaphragm, the heart, the great vessels, and the esophagus) may be at risk of possible injury during the chest drain insertion.
- The trocar technique, especially when performed in an emergency setting, is burdened by a high risk of possible complications.

INTRODUCTION

Chest drain placement is one of the most common surgical procedures performed in routine clinical practice. It can be done at the patient bedside, in the operating room, and in the emergency department, sometimes in life-threatening conditions (**Box 1**). The procedure is usually performed by thoracic surgeons, but, oftentimes, also by emergency physicians, intensivists, pulmonologists, interventional radiologists, and nonphysician advanced practitioners, in the emergency setting.[1,2] The thoracic drain evacuates air, blood, and fluids retained in the pleural cavity, monitors possible thoracic bleeding, prevents tension pneumothorax, enhances the lung reexpansion improving respiratory function and facilitates the postoperative recovery in patients submitted to thoracic/cardiac operations.

Despite the many benefits, chest tube insertion is not always a harmless procedure, and potential significant morbidity and mortality may exist. Collop and colleagues[3] reported a 3% early (generally drainage misplacement and pneumothorax) and 8% late complication rate (tube dislodgement and kinking, infection). Incorrect tube insertion also may have disastrous consequences: perforation of the right or left ventricle, of the main pulmonary artery, or the esophagus has in fact been described.

The aim of this article was to highlight the correct chest tube placement procedure and to focus on errors and clinical complications following its incorrect insertion into the chest.

---

[a] Department of Thoracic Surgery, University of Torino, Corso Dogliotti 14, Torino 10126, Italy; [b] Unit of Pulmonology, San Giovanni Battista Hospital, Via Genova, 3, Torino 10126, Italy
* Corresponding author.
E-mail address: pierluigi.filosso@unito.it

Thorac Surg Clin 27 (2017) 57–67
http://dx.doi.org/10.1016/j.thorsurg.2016.08.009

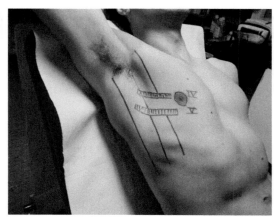

Fig. 1. The "safe triangle": where to correctly place a chest drain.

STANDARD SURGICAL TECHNIQUES FOR CHEST DRAIN PLACEMENT

The standard technique to correctly insert a chest drain is extensively described by the British Thoracic Surgery (BTS) guidelines.[4] Before proceeding to any invasive procedure, an exhaustive individual consent form, which explains the advantages and the possible complications of the surgical procedure, should be obtained from the patient and documented in the patient medical record.

The preferred patient's position should be supine, on the bed, slightly rotated, with the arm placed behind the head, to better expose the axillary area.

The drain should be inserted within the so-called "safe triangle," defined as the thoracic area between the latissimus dorsi muscle anterior edge, the pectoralis major muscle lateral edge, and a line superior to the horizontal level of the nipple with the apex below the axilla (**Fig. 1**). This area reduces the risk of injuring underlying vascular structures, such as the internal mammary artery, as well as to damage muscles or the breast, resulting also in a comfortable position for the patient.

In case of anterior or apical pneumothorax, a tube could be placed in the second intercostal space, in the mid clavicular line; however, this position may be dangerous and uncomfortable for the patient.

Particular care should be taken to drain pleural effusions or pneumothorax in a patient who previously underwent lung/cardiac surgery or pleurodesis (**Fig. 2**). These situations usually require exhaustive imaging studies. The diaphragm is in fact raised, as consequence of the former operation, and it could be injured during the tube placement; the lung also may present several dense adhesions and the risk of bleeding is therefore increased.

A different and lower tube position is required to drain fluid collection, especially loculated ones, as generally is observed as a consequence of a pleural empyema. Care should be taken to avoid diaphragm damage during the placement, or tube misplacement in the abdomen.

If a resident or a young physician places the tube, and the scheduled insertion should be outside the "triangle of safety," the procedure should be discussed with a senior surgeon. Both the National Patient Safety Agency (NPSA)[5] and BTS[4] guidelines recommend ultrasound guidance to insert a chest tube to drain fluid. Therefore, correct training in thoracic ultrasonography is required for the medical staff (senior and young physicians) involved in emergencies and in the care of patients with thoracic diseases.

Chest tubes are usually divided into *large bore* (≥20 F) and *small bore* (≤20 F) according to their size. French (F) is a standardized unit of measurement that was proposed by the French surgical instrument maker Joseph-Frederic-Benoit Charrière in 1860; F refers to the outer diameter of a cylindrical tube and is equivalent to 0.333 mm. The internal diameter (bore), which may vary according to the manufacturer and the length of the tube, is the

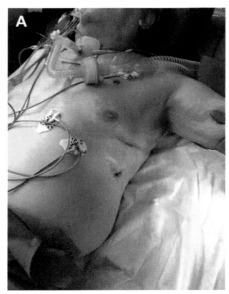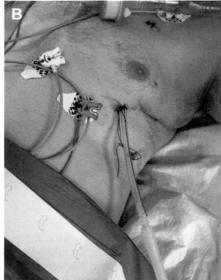

Fig. 2. Correct placement of a small-bore (20 F Argyle) chest drain for a residual pneumothorax after "uniportal" lung volume resection for severe emphysema. The tube is placed very close to the utility thoracotomy, not using the previous incision.

key determinant of pleural liquid (including blood and pus) flow through the drain. Therefore, the choice of the drain size must be based on the type of fluid to be drained from the pleural cavity.

Chest tubes may be placed either percutaneously (using a needle-introduced guide wire and/or an introducer sheath with a tract dilatator), by blunt dissection or by the trocar technique (**Fig. 3**). Usually, the percutaneous and the blunt dissection methods offer better control of the tube placement, and are the preferred approaches when a drain is placed "blindly." The patient's height and weight, anatomy, and chest habitus (anomalies/deformities) are also fundamental parameters to correctly choose the type of drain to be placed (**Fig. 4**). As reported in the literature, the trocar technique, compared with other less-invasive techniques, is burdened by a greater incidence of lung injuries.[6,7]

Regardless the adopted technique, the tube must be placed on the superior rib margin to avoid a possible injury to the intercostal neurovascular bundle; when the blunt dissection is used, the surgeon also should perform a finger sweep within the thoracic cavity, to confirm that the lung is not adherent to the chest wall, before introducing the drain.

Then, it is required to advance the tube far enough into the thorax so that its most peripheral hole (the so-called "sentinel hole") remains confined within the pleural space (**Fig. 5**).

The drain must be secured to the skin with a stitch, to avoid its possible dislodgement, especially if a prolonged duration is expected. A "u-stitch" should be placed around the tube thoracostomy during its placement: this stitch will then be tied down when the tube is removed, to close the skin incision.

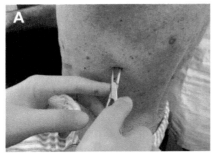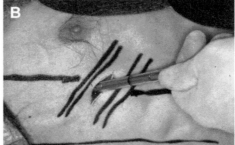

Fig. 3. Techniques for chest drain placement: (*A*) blunt technique; (*B*) trocar technique.

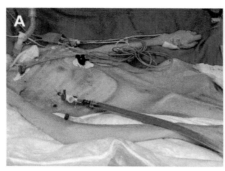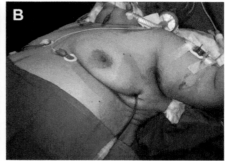

Fig. 4. Different chest drains according to the patient's body habitus: (*A*) small-bore catheter placed in a severely anorexic woman; (*B*) large-bore tube in an obese ventilated patient.

To assess its correct position and to prevent complications related to possible injuries of the anatomic structures in the proximity of the tube, a chest radiograph following the procedure is mandatory.[4] Another critical step following the procedure is to review both the preprocedural and postprocedural radiographic images to critically check clinical findings, such as residual pneumothorax, incompletely drained hemothorax, or pleural/mediastinal abnormalities, which may suggest possible iatrogenic injuries.

Despite the undoubted benefits of chest drainage, potential morbidity and mortality may be related to this procedure.

ERRORS AND COMPLICATIONS IN CHEST DRAIN INSERTION

Complications of the tube thoracostomy procedure may be categorized as acute, chronic, procedural, and nonprocedural.[8] The average complication rate after chest tube placement may vary between 5% and 10%.[9] The most frequently reported problems are tube malposition, other technical complications (1%), empyema (1%–2%), and bronchopleural fistula (rare).[8] Furthermore, any anatomic thoracic structure may be at risk during chest drainage insertion.

Although absolute contraindications to tube thoracostomy do not exist (especially in an emergency), one should be careful to place drains in immunocompromised patients, in those in whom a previous thoracic/cardiac operation (even transplantation) or pleurodesis have been performed, or in those with severe coagulopathy.[1]

Post drain placement complications also may be divided into early (occurring during the first 24–48 hours after tube placement) and chronic (occurring beyond this time).

Description of organ-specific complications will follow in this article.

INTRATHORACIC ORGANS INJURY
Lung Injury

The most common intrathoracic organ that may be injured is the lung. Pulmonary lacerations are more frequent in those patients who underwent a previous thoracic surgery or pleurodesis, in whom a high risk of dense adhesions is expected.[8] Particular care should be therefore taken in such patients and a careful thorough radiological examination is needed before chest tube insertion. Ultrasonography could be of great help to correctly delimitate pleural effusions before placing the tube. An intraparenchymal tube (**Fig. 6**) may lacerate the lung, causing bleeding and/or prolonged air leaks, may create a bronchopleural fistula, or lead to infection/lung abscess development. Hemorrhage is not always seen at the time of drain placement, but more frequently once it is removed. In case of severe and unresolved bleeding, immediate thoracotomy should be taken in consideration to repair the laceration.

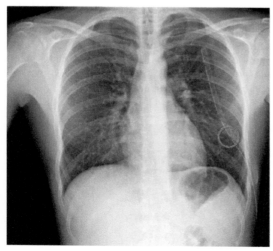

Fig. 5. Chest radiograph with left-side chest drain: the "sentinel hole" is correctly located into the thoracic cavity (*red circle*).

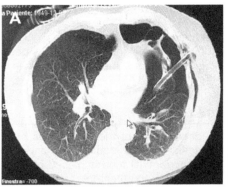
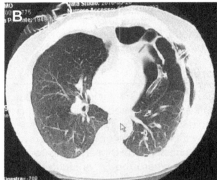

Fig. 6. Intraparenchymal chest tube placement (CT scan).

Diaphragmatic Injury

The low placement of the chest tube, just above the diaphragm, may result in diaphragm muscle dysfunction, perforation, or laceration. Diaphragmatic elevation is sometimes observed in large intra-abdominal neoplasms, ascites, obesity, and also late pregnancy. Furthermore, diaphragmatic acute/chronic hernia may increase the risk of muscle injury, especially if the trocar technique is used to introduce the drainage.

Cardiac and Great Vessel Injuries

Heart laceration after chest tube placement is a rare but not impossible condition (**Fig. 7**); this injury is often the consequence of the trocar technique used for the tube placement. Heart cavity penetration results in rapid blood output through the drainage, with associated catastrophic hemodynamic consequences.[8] The same dramatic impact is seen when the descending aorta is injured. Immediate thoracotomy with cardiopulmonary bypass is required to try to repair the laceration. Pulmonary and even subclavian artery injuries have been seldom reported[10–12]: an immediate thoracotomy was required also.

Mediastinal Injury

Even if rare, chest drainage abutting/trespassing the mediastinum has been occasionally reported.[13] The injury is usually caused by the placement of a large-bore chest tube using the trocar technique in patients who are hemodynamically unstable with severe chronic obstructive pulmonary disease with sudden development of pneumothorax (PNX), or in pulmonary contusions/hemothorax following blunt thoracic trauma. The tube may pass through the mediastinum, reaching the contralateral pleura, and it is well detected by a bedside chest radiograph. Gradual and careful removal of the tube is usually sufficient for the successful management of this condition.

Esophageal Injury

Esophageal injury due to chest tube placement is rare, and perforations have been described even in the case of a normal esophagus[14] or in various pathologic states, as well as in postesophageal surgery.[15,16] Mediastinum enlargement at chest radiograph and drainage of salivary or enteric liquids through the tube should raise suspicion of a possible esophageal laceration, but a radiological

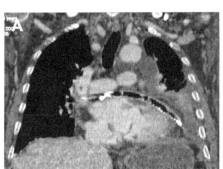
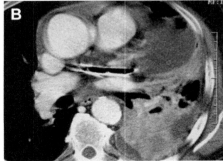

Fig. 7. (A, B) Heart injury after placement of a left-side chest drain using the trocar technique (CT scan).

confirmation is required, by performing a selected contrast study. An immediate surgical repair of the perforation, with the interposition of muscle or pleural flap is the mainstay of the treatment.

Horner Syndrome

The sympathetic trunk (ST) injury may cause Horner syndrome, characterized by miosis, ptosis, anhidrosis, and enophthalmos.[8] Horner syndrome, rarely caused by tube thoracostomy, may however occur when the chest drain is inserted up to the apex of the pleura, where the ST is located.[17,18] The mechanisms of injury may include direct sympathetic ganglion laceration, local inflammation, or fibrosis. A prompt clinical diagnosis and a subsequent appropriate repositioning of the chest tube may reduce the risk of permanent consequences.

INJURY OF EXTRATHORACIC ORGANS

Improper chest drain placement may result in an unintended intra-abdominal insertion; the incidence of such complication is very difficult to know, because most information is based on single case reports. The physicians should take care of the patient's body habitus (severely obese patients are, for example, at higher risk for tube malpositioning) and previous possible surgical interventions that could result in diaphragm elevation.

Gastric Injury

A direct injury of the stomach is rare in normal conditions, but it is more frequent when a wrong intra-abdominal tube is placed or in case of diaphragmatic acute/chronic laceration with abdominal viscera thoracic herniation,[19,20] a clinical condition that may mimic a pneumothorax.[21] A prompt surgical repair of the gastric laceration is therefore required.

Hepatic Injury

Bleeding from the tube and severe hemodynamic instability following right-sided tube thoracostomy should raise the suspicion of a possible hepatic injury (**Fig. 8**). This condition has been rarely

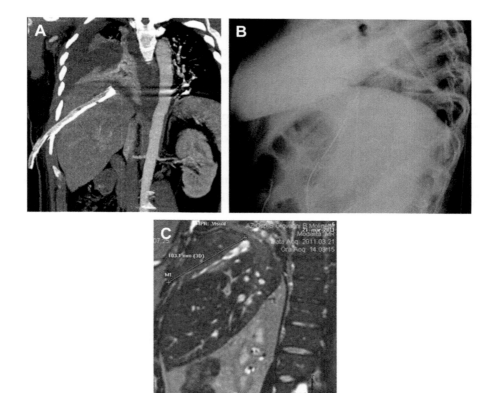

Fig. 8. Intrahepatic chest drain insertion following a blunt right-side pulmonary trauma. (*A*) CT scan. (*B*) PA chest radiograph. (*C*) Sagittal CT reconstruction. PA, postero-anterior.

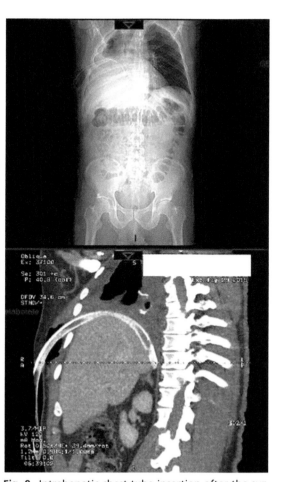

Fig. 9. Intrahepatic chest tube insertion after the surgical drainage of a right-side postpneumonectomy empyema cavity (CT scan).

reported in the literature,[22,23] however occurring principally in an emergency.

   The authors also observed an intrahepatic tube placement following the surgical drainage of a right postpneumonectomy empyema cavity

(**Fig. 9**): the intrahepatic tube was carefully removed and correctly replaced in the operating room. In general, the tube can be safely removed from the liver, but, due to the postremoval bleeding, hepatic embolization is sometimes required.[24,25]

Bowel Injury

Iatrogenic bowel injury following a chest drainage placement may occur in case of an acute/chronic diaphragmatic herniation through which the bowel is attracted into the thorax.[26] A prompt recognition of the clinical condition and a surgical repair are mandatory.

Splenic Injury

Splenic injuries after tube thoracostomy have been rarely reported[8,27,28]: bleeding through the tube is the immediate consequence of the laceration. In the literature, in one case the injury was managed by the insertion of fibrin sealant through the drainage tube, which was afterward successfully removed several days after; in a second case, a superficial splenic laceration occurred, but did not require any urgent surgical intervention. Moreover, the authors observed an unpublished case in which splenic injury occurred in a lung-transplanted patient after left tube thoracostomy for chronic hemothorax: an immediate laparotomy and splenectomy were necessary to control the bleeding.

OTHER COMPLICATIONS

Less severe complications of tube thoracostomy are described in the following sections.

Subcutaneous Placement

Sometimes the chest tube is placed outside the pleural space, in the subcutaneous tissue or within the muscular fibers in an emergency and/or by nonexperienced physicians (**Fig. 10**).

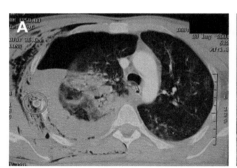
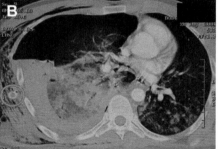

Fig. 10. Extrathoracic (*red circle*) chest drain inserted after a severe chest trauma (CT scan).

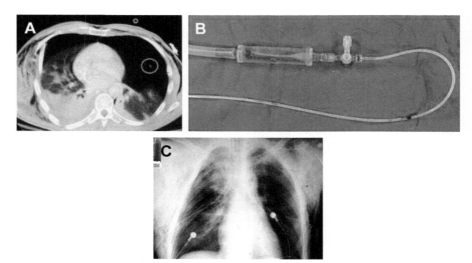

Fig. 11. An example of wrong chest tube size. Severe chest trauma. (*A*) The patient presented with bilateral pneumothorax, pulmonary contusion, and right-sided hemothorax. He required rapid intubation in the field and was transported to the nearest hospital by helicopter. The left pneumothorax was drained using a small-bore drain (Pleurocath) (*B*) (*red circle* in *A*), connected to a Heimlich valve. At the arrival at the hospital he was drained with 2 large-bore chest tubes. (*C*) Postdrainage chest radiograph with satisfactory pulmonary reexpansion.

The suspicion of tube misplacement should rise when it does not evacuate air or fluid. Some patients (severely obese, multiple rib fractures) seem to be at higher risk for this complication. A prompt control with a chest radiograph following the procedure can confirm its wrong positioning, in which case its replacement is required.

Miscellaneous Issues

Figs. 11 and **12** show some examples of errors in site and size of chest drains. In particular, small-bore chest tubes are sometimes used in an emergency setting to drain air or blood after severe thoracic trauma, but are incorrectly placed, resulting ineffective. Malignant pleural effusions in critically patients are occasionally managed with small-bore tubes under ultrasonographic guidance; slurry talc poudrage through such drains is then performed. In many occasions (especially by nonexperienced physicians) the tube is placed too basal, close to the diaphragm (**Fig. 13**) resulting effective to drain the fluid, but inappropriate for pleurodesis.

Chest tube dislodgement (**Fig. 14**) usually occurs in case of small-bore tubes and prolonged

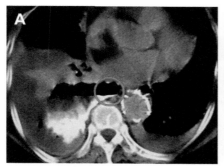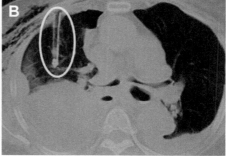

Fig. 12. An example of wrong chest drain site. (*A*) Boerhaave syndrome CT with contrast. Contrast expands in the right pleural space trough an esophageal laceration (*red circle*). (*B*) The chest drain was incorrectly placed anteriorly (*yellow circle*), unable to drain the pleural fluid.

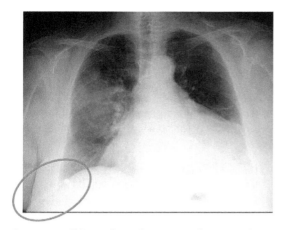

Fig. 13. Small-bore chest drain wrongly inserted in a patient with right-sided malignant pleural effusion; the drain is too basal and very close to the diaphragm (*red circle*), Slurry talc poudrage through the tube was ineffective.

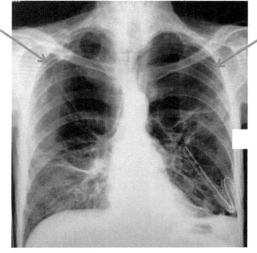

Fig. 15. Left-sided chest tube placed for secondary pneumothorax, with double kinking. Red arrows show the large apical bilateral bullae.

duration (weeks). Moreover, the necessary changes of the patient's position by the nursing staff (especially in the intensive care unit), may result in drainage dislodgement. Infection of the insertion point is also frequent, requiring tube removal and its replacement.

Intrathoracic drainage malposition is frequently observed in emergency, when the tube is placed in hurried and less controlled conditions, especially using the trocar technique. The drainage results in insufficient/poor drainage or initial good and later poor drainage of air, blood, or other fluids. Thoracic computed tomography (CT) is considered the most effective imaging tool to check the correct drainage intrathoracic position,

also assessing possible misplacement (intraparenchymal, intrafissural, mediastinal locations).[29,30]

The presence of dense adhesions or large bullae may divert the correct tube proceeding into the pleural cavity, resulting in drainage kinking (**Fig. 15**).

Finally, the occurrence of drainage fragmentation and possible intrathoracic retention is a rare occurrence,[31,32] but more frequent for thin small-bore catheters. The authors have had the experience of 2 cases of Pleurocath (Prodimed, Neuilly-en-Thelle, France) drains that ruptured after their prolonged duration, in which thoracoscopy was required to remove the retained fragment (**Fig. 16**).

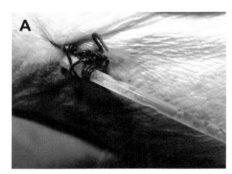
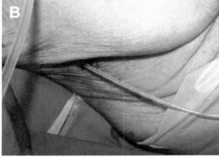

Fig. 14. (*A, B*) Dislodgement of small-bore drains (Pleurocath) after several days of in situ stay. In both cases, the drain holes are outside the chest.

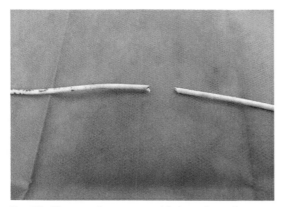

Fig. 16. Pleurocath rupture with intrathoracic retention, which required thoracoscopy to remove the fragment (surgical specimen).

SUMMARY

In conclusion, tube thoracostomy is one of the most common invasive procedures in hospitalized patients; correct indication, caliber, and proper insertion of the chest tube is of paramount importance. The surgical maneuver is not always devoid of complications, and potential significant morbidity and mortality may exist. Moreover, inappropriately positioned drains may be unapparent clinically in the short term, but may have serious outcomes in the long term. The use of ultrasonography has demonstrated to reduce the risk of errors in the tube insertion, especially when limited fluid/air collections have to be drained.

Every physician potentially involved in a thoracic drainage placement should take into account benefits and complications inherent to this invasive procedure, which may seriously affect patients' course and outcomes.

REFERENCES

1. Gilbert TB, McGrath BJ, Soberman M. Chest tubes: indications, placement, management, and complications. J Intensive Care Med 1993;8:73–86.
2. Barton ED, Epperson M, Hoyt DB, et al. Prehospital needle aspiration and tube thoracostomy in trauma victims: a six-year experience with aeromedical crews. J Emerg Med 1995;13:155–63.
3. Collop NA, Kim S, Sahn SA. Analysis of tube thoracostomy performed by pulmonologists at a teaching hospital. Chest 1997;112:709–13.
4. Laws D, Neville E, Duffy J, Pleural Diseases Group, Standards of Care Committee, British Thoracic Society. BTS guidelines for the insertion of a chest drain. Thorax 2003;58(Suppl II):ii53–9.
5. Available at: www.npsa.nhs.uk/alerts-and-directives/rapidrr/risks -of-chest-drain-insertion/.
6. Helling TS, Gyles NR 3rd, Eisenstein CL, et al. Complications following blunt and penetrating injuries in 216 victims of chest trauma requiring tube thoracostomy. J Trauma 1989;29:1367–70.
7. Deneuville M. Morbidity of percutaneous tube thoracostomy in trauma patients. Eur J Cardiothorac Surg 2002;22:673–8.
8. Kwiatt M, Tarbox A, Seamon MJ, et al. Thoracostomy tubes: a comprehensive review of complications and related topics. Int J Crit Illn Inj Sci 2014; 4:143–55.
9. Bailey RC. Complications of tube thoracostomy in trauma. J Accid Emerg Med 2000;17:111–4.
10. Gabriel CA, Adama DP, Salmane BP, et al. A case report of iatrogenic pulmonary artery injury due to chest-tube insertion repaired under cardiopulmonary bypass. Case Rep Med 2013;2013:590971.
11. Taub PJ, Lajam F, Kim U. Erosion into the subclavian artery by a chest tube. J Trauma 1999;47:972–4.
12. Moskal TL, Liscum KR, Mattox KL. Subclavian artery obstruction by tube thoracostomy. J Trauma 1997; 43:368–9.
13. Chen YF, Chen CY, Hsu CL, et al. Malpositioning of the chest tube across the anterior mediastinum is risky in chronic obstructive pulmonary disease patients with pneumothorax. Interact Cardiovasc Thorac Surg 2011;13:109–11.
14. Shapira OM, Aldea GS, Kupferschmid J, et al. Delayed perforation of the esophagus by a closed thoracostomy tube. Chest 1993;104:1897–8.
15. Adebonojo SA. Delayed perforation of the esophagus by a closed thoracostomy tube. Chest 1994; 106:1306.
16. Johnson JF, Wright DR. Chest tube perforation of esophagus following repair of esophageal atresia. J Pediatr Surg 1990;25:1227–30.
17. Baird R, Al-Balushi Z, Wackett J, et al. Iatrogenic Horner syndrome after tube thoracostomy. J Pediatr Surg 2009;44:2012–4.
18. Thomas DT, Dagli TE, Kiyan G. Horner's syndrome as a rare complication of tube thoracostomy: case reports and review of literature. J Pediatr Surg 2013;48:1429–33.
19. Zieren J, Enzweiler C, Müller JM. Tube thoracostomy complicates unrecognized diaphragmatic rupture. Thorac Cardiovasc Surg 1999;47:199–202.
20. Andrabi SA, Andrabi SL, Mansha M, et al. An iatrogenic complication of closed tube thoracostomy for penetrating chest trauma. N Z Med J 2007;120: U2784.
21. Yilmaz M, Isik B, Ara C. Gastric perforation during chest tube placement for acute diaphragmatic rupture and review of the literature. Injury Extra 2006;37:71–5.
22. Harte S, Casey RG, Mannion D, et al. When is a pneumothorax not a pneumothorax? J Pediatr Surg 2005;40:586–7.

23. Tanaka S, Hirohashi K, Uenishi T, et al. Surgical repair of a liver injury in a patient: accompanied with tricuspid regurgitation. Hepatogastroenterology 2003;50:523–5.

24. Tait P, Waheed U, Bell S. Successful removal of mal-positioned chest drain within the liver by emboliza-tion of the transhepatic track. Cardiovasc Intervent Radiol 2009;32:825–7.

25. Hegarty C, Gerstenmaier JF, Brophy D. "Chest tube" removal after liver transgression. J Vasc Interv Ra-diol 2012;23:275.

26. Collazo E, Díaz Iglesias C. Iatrogenic perforation of the intrathoracic colon after a late traumatic dia-phragmatic hernia. Rev Esp Enferm Dig 1994;86:767–70 [in Spanish].

27. Darragh L, Clements WDB. An unusual iatrogenic splenic injury managed conservatively. Inj Extra 2011;42:58–9.

28. Schmidt U, Stalp M, Gerich T, et al. Chest tube decompression of blunt chest injuries by physicians in the field: effectiveness and complications. J Trauma 1998;44:98–101.

29. Cameron EW, Mirvis SE, Shanmuganathan K, et al. Computed tomography of malpositioned thoracos-tomy drains: a pictorial essay. Clin Radiol 1997;52:187–93.

30. Lim KE, Tai SC, Chan CY, et al. Diagnosis of malpo-sitioned chest tubes after emergency tube thoracos-tomy: is computed tomography more accurate than chest radiograph? Clin Imaging 2005;29:401–5.

31. Paddle A, Elahi M, Newcomb A. Retained foreign body following pleural drainage with a small-bore catheter. Gen Thorac Cardiovasc Surg 2010;58:42–4.

32. Cunningham JP, Knott EM, Gasior AC, et al. Is routine chest radiograph necessary after chest tube removal? J Pediatr Surg 2014;49:1493–5.

Index

Note: Page numbers of article titles are in **boldface** type.

Moving?

Make sure your subscription moves with you!

To notify us of your new address, find your **Clinics Account Number** (located on your mailing label above your name), and contact customer service at:

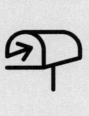

Email: journalscustomerservice-usa@elsevier.com

800-654-2452 (subscribers in the U.S. & Canada)
314-447-8871 (subscribers outside of the U.S. & Canada)

Fax number: 314-447-8029

Elsevier Health Sciences Division
Subscription Customer Service
3251 Riverport Lane
Maryland Heights, MO 63043

ELSEVIER

Printed and bound by CPI Group (UK) Ltd, Croydon, CR0 4YY

08/05/2025

01864696-0009